T0342359

Also available in the Sociology of Health Professions series

Professional Health Regulation in the Public Interest
International Perspectives
Edited by **John Martyn Chamberlain, Mike Dent and Mike Saks**

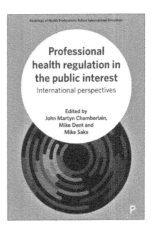

"With enormous variation in the delivery of healthcare, how it is regulated is more important than ever. The authors herein dissect the differences and enlighten us with forensic ability over a global range."
John Flood, Griffith University Law School

HB $75.00 ISBN 9781447332268
288 pages June 2018

For more information about the series visit
bristoluniversitypress.co.uk/sociology-of-health-professions

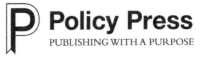

SUPPORT WORKERS AND THE HEALTH PROFESSIONS IN INTERNATIONAL PERSPECTIVE

The Invisible Providers of Health Care

Edited by
Mike Saks

First published in Great Britain in 2020 by

Policy Press
University of Bristol
1-9 Old Park Hill
Bristol
BS2 8BB
UK
t: +44 (0)117 954 5940
pp-info@bristol.ac.uk
www.policypress.co.uk

© Policy Press 2020

British Library Cataloguing in Publication Data
A catalogue record for this book is available from the British Library

ISBN 978-1-4473-5210-5 hardcover
ISBN 978-1-4473-5212-9 ePub
ISBN 978-1-4473-5211-2 ePdf

Cover design by Cube
Front cover image: iStock-522116113
Printed and bound in Great Britain by CPI Group (UK) Ltd,
Croydon, CR0 4YY
Policy Press uses environmentally responsible print partners

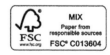

Contents

Notes on contributors

Editor

Mike Saks is Emeritus Professor at the University of Suffolk, having previously been Research Professor in Health Policy there. He is also Visiting Professor at the University of Lincoln, the Royal Veterinary College, University of London, and the University of Westminster in the UK, and the University of Toronto in Canada. He has served on the Executive Boards of six universities, including as Chief Executive, and acted as a chair/member of the NHS and other health committees at all levels. He has also been an advisor to governments and professional bodies internationally in health and social care and made many keynote presentations – having published some 20 books and 100 articles/book chapters in his specialist areas of health, professions and regulation from a sociological and wider social science perspective. These publications and presentations have included those on health support work, an area in which he has directly contributed to government policy in Canada and the UK. He was a recent President of the International Sociological Association Research Committee on Professional Groups and is the current Vice President of the International Sociological Association Research Committee on the Sociology of Health, which both support the Policy Press series on the Sociology of Health Professions: Future International Directions, of which this book is a part. He is also a member of the Editorial/International Advisory Board of several international journals, including the *Journal of Professions and Organization* (Oxford University Press). Most recently he has become Honorary Senior Advisor to the United Nations on public sector leadership and is a founder member of the United Nations-sponsored Institute for Responsible Leadership.

Other contributors

Judith Allsop is Visiting Professor of Health Policy, School of Social and Political Sciences, University of Lincoln, UK.

Joana Almeida is Lecturer in the Department of Applied Social Studies, University of Bedfordshire, UK.

Nelson Barros is Associate Professor of Sociology, Faculty of Medicine, Campinas University, Brazil.

Whitney Berta is Associate Professor, Institute of Health Policy, Management and Evaluation, University of Toronto, Canada.

Adrian Rohit Dass is a doctoral student, Institute of Health Policy, Management and Evaluation, University of Toronto, Canada.

Raisa Deber is Professor of Health Policy, Institute of Health Policy, Management and Evaluation, University of Toronto, Canada.

Mike Dent is Emeritus Professor of Health Care Organisation, Staffordshire University, UK.

Anna Dunér is Professor and Deputy Head of the Department of Social Work, University of Gothenburg, Sweden.

Miwako Hosoda is Professor and Vice President, Seisa University, Japan.

Audrey Laporte is Associate Professor of Health Economics, Institute of Health Policy, Management and Evaluation, University of Toronto, Canada.

Aukje Leemeijer is Senior Lecturer, HAN University of Applied Sciences in Nijmegen and a doctoral student, Utrecht School of Governance, Utrecht University, The Netherlands.

Andreas Liljegren is Senior Researcher in Social Work, University of Gothenburg, Sweden.

Janet M. Lum is Professor, Department of Politics and Public Administration, Ryerson University, Canada.

Susan Nancarrow is Emeritus Professor, Southern Cross University, Australia.

Mirko Noordegraaf is Professor of Public Management, Utrecht School of Governance and Vice Dean for Societal Impact, Faculty of Law, Economics and Governance, Utrecht University, The Netherlands.

Elisabeth Olin is Professor and Head of the Department of Social Work, University of Gothenburg, Sweden.

A. Paul Williams is Emeritus Professor, Institute of Health Policy, Management and Evaluation, University of Toronto, Canada.

Katherine Zagrodney is a doctoral student, Institute of Health Policy, Management and Evaluation, University of Toronto, Canada.

Editors' overview

This edited text is the second in a series entitled the *Sociology of Health Professions: Future International Directions*, published by Policy Press and edited by Mike Saks and Mike Dent, supported by a high-profile international advisory board. The research-based series is focused on giving innovatory sociological insights into the past, present and future development of the health professions. It is mainly oriented towards final year and postgraduate students, academic lecturers/researchers, practitioners and policy makers. In filling a major gap in the literature as the first social scientific text on the role of support workers operating with health professions in the provision of health care, it is resonant with the template for the general Policy Press series on the sociology of the health professions in that it aims:

- to inform and stimulate debate about issues in the sociology of health professions;
- to influence policy development and practice in the fields concerned;
- to make a significant contribution to academic thinking in the sociology of health; and
- to produce original national/international work of high quality.

The significance of the current volume on *Support Workers and the Health Professions in International Perspective: The Invisible Providers of Health Care* is underlined by the need to give more attention to health support workers in light of their growing importance in working with health professions in providing health care in Western societies and beyond. The special significance of this collection, introduced by Mike Saks as editor, is that the various expert contributions assembled here come together as part of the inaugural social science book on support workers operating in conjunction with health professions in health care, which has ramifications for all modern societies. As such, with both substantial academic and regulatory and other policy implications, it fits well into the Policy Press series on the sociology of the health professions. This is the second book in the series following the first, edited by John Martyn Chamberlain, Mike Dent and Mike Saks, on *Professional Health Regulation in the Public Interest: International Perspectives*. More commissioned work in the series is to come in the near future on subjects such as the allied health professions, dentistry and medical policy in an international context.

Mike Saks and Mike Dent

ONE

Introduction: Support workers and the health professions

Mike Saks

Introduction

The book examines the role of support workers, particularly in their interface with the health professions. This disparate, but very large, group of workers is defined by providing face-to-face care and other support of a personal or confidential nature to service users in a variety of settings. However, crucially, they do not hold qualifications accredited by a professional association and are not typically formally regulated by a professional body (Saks and Allsop 2007). The volume is original as there are no known books to date that analyse from a sociological or wider social science perspective the role of support workers in the health care labour force in these or other terms. This edited collection attempts to do just that from a largely neo–Weberian theoretical perspective which examines professions in terms of the various forms of social closure that they have gained in a competitive market, underwritten by the state – based on legally underpinned and exclusionary registers of practitioners protecting them against outsiders (Saks 2010). The achievement of this position, which brings privileges of income, status and power to insiders, is seen as being linked to the interests of players in such top-dog occupations. Although neo–Weberian writers have been criticised in practice for not giving sufficient attention to non-professional workers in their analyses of professionalisation (Saks 2016a), this volume puts such groups centre stage, including in their relationship to professions.

The focus here, though, is on the health arena – in particular on research on various aspects of the operation of the huge cohort of health support workers who are critical providers of health care globally. In so doing, the book takes an international perspective drawing on illustrations from several modern neo-liberal countries, spanning from the UK, The Netherlands, Portugal and Sweden through Japan and Australia to Brazil and Canada. As such, it variously examines the relationship of such relatively invisible workers with the myriad of health professions which sit at a variety of levels in the pecking order. At the top of the hierarchy concerned is the medical profession, which has tended to dominate the field internationally and has a directive role in health care (Saks 2015), followed by historically subordinated groups like nurses (Borsay and Hunter 2012) and allied health professionals with limited jurisdiction such as dieticians and physiotherapists (Larkin 2002). Social workers are also included in this analysis in the book in so far as they can be conceptualised as part of a caring profession operating within wider definitions of health and wellbeing, with a direct impact on quality of life in such areas as mental health and disability (Lishman et al 2018).

Drawing on a number of experts in the field, the book provides a novel analysis of support workers – who have their own layers of complexity, ranging as they do from care assistants and complementary and alternative therapists to occupational therapy and physiotherapy aides (Saks et al 2000). They have largely lacked transparency to health researchers and policy makers alike, even though they characteristically make up by far the greatest proportion of the health labour force in modern societies (see, for example, Dubois et al 2006). Despite their relative invisibility, health support workers are vitally important to enhancing health in the long-term future, another unique aspect that is underlined in this book. As such, their numbers are fast growing as modern governments strive to combat illness in the most cost effective manner in a world of finite resources – not least with the rapidly expanding prevalence of chronic conditions with an ageing population and a necessarily restricted number of fully-fledged, but much more expensive, health professional workers like doctors and less well paid and lower status nurses, members of the allied health professions and social workers (World Health Organization 2019).

Taking the concept of health in its widest sense, this volume therefore situates support workers in the wider health care division of labour – covering a broad span of paid support personnel in addition to similarly highly-valued volunteers and carers in the private and public sector. It does so by considering the development of the diverse range of health support workers in the context of their evolving relationship to the health professionals whom they so frequently work alongside and/or to whom they report. Since many support workers operate independently in people's own homes and statutory registers for them do not generally exist, there can be greater risks to clients from support workers than health personnel on professional registers in more formal organisational settings in both commercialised and non-commercialised areas (Saks et al 2000). Such regulatory risks are centrally examined in this book, alongside the working conditions of health support personnel. The book also gives central consideration to the challenges and opportunities presented by the employment of such workers in the community, hospital, residential and other institutional settings on a devolved, complementary or labour substitution basis. This and other considerations cover the part played by health support workers and their interplay with health professions in an international context, including their management and leadership. This introduction now turns to elaborate in more detail the contributory chapters of this book – each of which looks at a different dimension of health support work.

Contributions to the book

Following Chapter one, which throws into focus the main themes of the book, the analysis of health support workers in the labour market begins with Chapter two by Mike Saks and Katherine Zagrodney on 'Health professions, support workers and the precariat'. This considers from a neo-Weberian theoretical perspective whether they can be seen as part of the new precariat as neo-Marxist writers have suggested – in a more fundamental fashion than has increasingly been ascribed to health professions themselves. Examining the working conditions of health support workers in the health care division of labour, this novel chapter is based empirically on the parallel cases of the UK and Canada, with which the authors are very familiar. It concludes that such trends are exaggerated. Despite the wide gulf in working conditions that continues to exist between this group and health professional occupations, and the precarious conditions of many health support workers, the heterogeneous position of such workers in the labour market is felt to militate against an all-encompassing theoretical approach – especially in relation to the development of a self-conscious and cohesive class as envisaged by some neo-Marxists. The chapter concludes by discussing the various policy implications that arise from this analysis.

Chapter three by Paul Williams and Janet Lum on 'Unpaid informal carers: The "shadow" workforce in health care' is a reminder that, in considering an invisible workforce in health care, we also need to factor in the vast army of unpaid, little trained and largely unregulated informal carers – alongside the ranks of health support workers. Both have been neglected in the focus of much of the international literature on highly trained, regulated and visible health professionals that have achieved exclusionary social closure in neo-Weberian terms. In the case of informal carers, these include family, friends and neighbours who deliver a significant proportion of everyday care to support the wellbeing and independence of increasing numbers of people facing multiple chronic health and social needs. This chapter charts the characteristics and contributions of informal carers with particular reference to Canada and examines why they are currently attracting so much attention. It also underlines the challenges faced by such carers as they deal with a growing burden of caring for the increasing numbers of people with complex needs in an ageing population. A key issue for policy makers is therefore how best to support them without excessively pushing up costs, as the emphasis shifts from institutional to community care. The chapter finishes by showcasing new initiatives that are engaging multi-generations, businesses, communities and cities in redefining caregiving.

Mike Dent in Chapter four writes on 'The management and leadership of support workers', with a focus on the UK and the broader European setting. As part of this, he examines from a neo-Weberian perspective the development of the management and organisation of health and social care support work following the introduction of the New Public Management. He illustrates this with reference to the redefinition of the professional jurisdiction of the nursing profession in the final decades of the 20th century. Concerns over the management and organisation of support workers under the New Public Management has more recently resulted in greater emphasis being given to professional regulation and leadership in a management discourse, within the framework of the New Public Governance. He argues that this has led support workers to become more professionalised to increase management effectiveness. While this move has to date fallen short of attaining classic neo-Weberian exclusionary social closure, it has importantly meant that support workers are increasingly recruited with appropriate values to deliver on the new agenda of 'responsibilisation'.

Meanwhile, Chapter five by Mike Saks and Judith Allsop is entitled 'Regulation, risk and health support work'. It starts by discussing the limited regulation of support workers as compared to health professionals from a neo-Weberian viewpoint. The ensuing risks are then highlighted, drawing on the illustrative example of the UK, and especially England given the different political paths taken by its increasingly devolved constituent countries. The authors claim that it may be in the public interest, in terms of protecting service users and their carers, to extend the existing regulatory framework in a number of modern societies. The need for this is seen as being accentuated by the increasing challenge that health professions have faced in the wake of publicity given to the escalating number of adverse events. In order to mitigate risk, it is argued that consideration should be given to extending state regulatory controls, establishing occupational registers, increasing employer and professional managerial controls in the public and private sector, and implementing additional requirements for continuing educational development. Health support workers, who are numerically by far the largest group of paid health personnel, are felt to remain both under regulated and under researched. Nonetheless, from a policy viewpoint, it is vital that there is not only more protection for clients and their surrounding networks, but also of vulnerable health support workers themselves.

In Chapter six Susan Nancarrow considers 'The interface of health support workers with the allied health professions', this time with a comparative focus on Australia and the UK. She begins by describing the allied health workforce, before exploring the consequent evolution of the support workforce linked to the allied health professions – not least by examining the reasons for the growth of this support workforce, the contexts in which it is used, the negotiation of its boundaries, and the challenges and opportunities it raises. This chapter claims that the heterogeneous allied health support workforce has developed through two models, each with different types of workers. The first is the profession-led model, based on the neo-Weberian concept of the professional project, in which allied health professions introduced support roles to expand and maintain their market monopoly and autonomy in key areas. The second is the managerial model, which instead privileges the 'patient–centred' goals of increasing role flexibility by recognising and rewarding individuals' skills and competencies and working across traditional professional and organisational boundaries. The chapter concludes by outlining some of the key challenges faced by the allied health support workforce in this context in the future.

Chapter seven by Andreas Liljegren, Anna Dunér and Elisabeth Olin is entitled 'Support workers in social care: Between social work professionals and service users'. The authors redress the balance in the volume by examining current debates about the role of support workers in social care in Sweden specifically. They explore whether the support worker service should be run by staff or by the users within a neo-Weberian perspective. As such, they describe and analyse the role of support workers for disabled people in two settings – support workers in residential social care and personal assistants in domiciliary care, both operating within Swedish social work. The two settings are shown to have organised social care in radically different manners in terms of power relations. As such, residential care workers chose a traditional path with staff subordinating service users by claiming to be experts in helping. However, the personal assistants took a more unorthodox direction by themselves being subordinated to service users. Both of these groups might be seen as a new precariat in social care because of their working conditions, but this case raises the question of how best to address social care issues at a national political level – a question that can also be posed in other societies.

In Chapter eight Aukje Leemeijer and Mirko Noordegraaf, in a very topical contribution, write on 'Health professionals and peer support workers in mental health settings', using The Netherlands as an illustrative focus. They note that an increasing trend in many Western countries is for mental health institutions to employ 'peer support workers' as co-workers in professional teams. Peer support workers are clients or former clients in mental health care who are trained and educated to transform their personal experience into 'experiential knowledge' to help improve 'client centredness'. However, using a neo-Weberian approach, they indicate that the rise of peer support workers is not undisputed and mental health professionals – psychiatrists, psychologists, nurses and therapists – show ambivalent responses. The experiential knowledge of peer support workers may challenge the status and dominance of traditional expert knowledge and influence professional powers and identities. This challenge is held to be strengthened by the potential of peer support workers themselves to professionalise and the influence of institutional surroundings, including how peer support workers and service organisations deal with risks and accountability. This analysis has significant policy implications for the interweaving of new forms of knowledge in support work.

Chapter nine features Joana Almeida and Nelson Barros considering 'Complementary and alternative medicine as an invisible health support workforce'. They argue that in ageing Western societies where chronic conditions have become more prevalent, complementary and alternative medicine (CAM) practices and practitioners have assumed an important role in areas such as health promotion, rehabilitation, and compassionate, preventative and palliative care. Yet collaborative partnerships between CAM practitioners, other professionally qualified health care workers and the state have rarely materialised. By using the neo-Weberian social closure theory of the professions, this chapter examines how far CAM practitioners have formed part of a precarious and undervalued health support workforce, in an analysis centred on the interlinked societies of Brazil and Portugal. It is suggested that CAM practitioners have in a number of respects resembled health support workers, especially in their statutorily unregulated status and/

or subordinated role to the medical profession. Nonetheless, it is not a perfect fit. In Brazil CAM practices, but not CAM practitioners, are statutorily regulated, while in Portugal CAM practitioners are statutorily regulated, although they remain marginalised. It is concluded that CAM practitioners have largely been an invisible health support workforce, despite increasing public sympathy and legitimation from the World Health Organization.

In Chapter ten Audrey Laporte, Adrian Rohit Dass, Whitney Berta, Raisa Deber and Katherine Zagrodney explore 'Personal support workers and the labour market', centred on a case study of Canada. Their team-based analysis of personal support workers (PSWs) – as they are known in Canada – suggests from a neo-Weberian perspective that, while it is helpful to consider the PSW labour market as a whole, it is better thought of as a series of sub-markets which comprise the hospital, long-term care, and home and community care sectors. These sectors may differ in terms of such factors as wages, benefits, hours worked and working conditions, as well as in the socio-demographic characteristics of PSWs working in each of the sectors. Given that sectoral differences in PSW characteristics affect labour supply behaviours and outcomes – as, for example, in creating differences in the proportion of PSWs nearing retirement age – it is emphasised that awareness of the heterogeneous nature of the PSW labour market is an important consideration in resource planning. The chapter also explores how PSWs compare to other health professions such as nursing, and makes select references to the international PSW literature in charting a course forward.

Finally, Miwako Hosoda brings the volume to a close in Chapter eleven by contributing on 'The role of health support workers in the ageing crisis', very appropriately situating her account in Japan – which contains the world's longest-living population. Having said this, developing an adequate care system with health support workers to meet the needs of the elderly is a global issue. In Japan family members previously cared for the elderly and those with disabilities. However, as the author notes, today the roles of families have changed, and care is more frequently provided by non-family members. As a result, the long-term care insurance system was implemented in 2000. Under this system, certain services are provided by qualified professional health care staff as defined in classic neo-Weberian terms. However, to realise an appropriate quality of life for older people and those with disabilities, more services than those provided by the long-term care insurance are often required. This results in additional services being performed by non-professional health support workers and home helpers. The chapter raises concerns about female labour with low wages and the practice of health and medical care by unqualified persons. On the other hand, this type of personalised care can provide a higher quality of life for the elderly and people with disabilities. This may be helped by a number of initiatives, including tailored educational and immigration programmes. As such, Japan may be a crucial testing ground for potential solutions to the ageing crisis as far as health support workers are concerned.

Key overarching messages

This summary of the individual chapter contributions to this edited book crystallises its main features which include, among others: highlighting the key role of support workers in relation to users and their carers internationally in the ever-changing socio-political and demographic environment of neo-liberal societies; examining theoretically and empirically their relationship with various layers of health professions; considering regulatory matters associated with support workers in different settings; and enhancing our understanding of the location of support workers in the wider labour market. The contributors were carefully chosen and briefed to provide a cohesive overall approach to health support workers and their interface with the health professions, albeit with each author in this edited collection dealing with different and complementary facets of the agenda. The overarching integration comes through the interpenetrating nature of the various offerings, covering a wide range of support worker occupations and issues in modern societies. So what key messages can be drawn from this volume?

What overridingly comes out of the book as highlighted by Chapter two by Saks and Zagrodney and Chapter ten by Laporte and colleagues is that support workers operating beneath the authority of the professions are generally less well rewarded in the labour market in a comparative material sense. In addition, as Williams and Lum underline in Chapter three, we ignore at our peril their relationship to the huge army of unpaid caregivers in this equation. As regards paid support workers, various chapters demonstrate there is a degree of variation in their working conditions and activities in different organisations and in the home and community sector, despite such potentially unifying developments as increased training and education or indeed the implementation of the New Public Management and, more recently, the New Public Governance as flagged in Chapter four by Dent. This applies too to the relationship of support workers to a broad span of health and care professions who may at times view them as an encroaching threat to their self-interests, while also seeing them on other occasions as a helpful mechanism in devolving 'dirty work' to enhance their professional standing. This is made especially clear in Chapters six to eight by Nancarrow, Liljegren, Dunér and Olin, and Leemeijer and Noordegraaf respectively who highlight the relevance of this interest-based dynamic in various international contexts.

There is a clear contrast in the position of most support workers to that of the health professions which – for all their failings as accentuated by recent scandals – have typically followed other professions in being able to command more lucrative and regularised positions within the societies in which they are employed. This has built on the exclusionary social closure that they have developed and the consequent emergence of professional associations (Flood 2018). As Chapter five by Saks and Allsop suggests in the UK, health support workers may pose a higher level of risk as compared to health professions in relation to their clients – as they may need a greater degree of regulatory mitigation to protect users of their services. This is particularly accentuated as their role expands with rising levels of longstanding conditions linked to the further extension of the life span as exemplified *in extremis* by Hosoda in Chapter eleven in the case of Japan. These are not, though, segmented agendas; as Chapter five accentuates, health professions such as nursing are increasingly taking on oversight roles in relation to support workers, which has served to stiffen public protection. This does not of course apply to a large number of support worker roles. This is illustrated by the marginalised case of complementary and alternative medicine explored in Chapter nine by Almeida and Barros. They make clear that there is a less straight forward relationship of this heterogeneous group of practitioners to the classic definition of support work in Brazil and Portugal, albeit for rather different regulatory reasons.

However, there have been changes in the health care division of labour. The shifting position of health professions in this context can perhaps best be depicted metaphorically as moving from a zoo, where independent self-regulating professions construct their own self-regulatory cages, to a circus, where the state as ringmaster seeks to exert greater control of their operation in an era of 'regulatory self-regulation' (Chamberlain 2015). This is how Saks (2016b) describes the recent transition of the English medical profession, although he notes that the environment has recently become more akin to a safari park in which different types of health and care professions have been encouraged by government to work together, as opposed to delivering in a series of silos. In terms of metaphors, Saks (2015) has also pertinently described the health support worker milieu as akin to the Wild West. The Wild West popularly refers to the period in the second half of the 19th century in the United States when there was little law and order. At this time bandits, outlaws and others ran wild to the detriment of local populations. The Wild West was ultimately tamed by regulation. This involved the establishment of government through, among other things, the appointment of sheriffs and deputies who managed to reduce lawlessness to the benefit of the wider public (Nolan 2003). There are parallels with the current support worker workforce in many neo-liberal societies – they are the often invisible providers of the bulk of hands-on health care who demand further regulatory attention from the state and employers in protecting the public, not least in terms of their fast growing significance in the health division of labour.

It is not therefore surprising that a further central agenda of the various chapters considered in this book has been to make recommendations on international policy directions in relation to health support workers in future. This encompasses both the public and private sector as support workers are increasingly involved in health care, in association with health professionalised groups such as doctors, midwives and nurses. In this light, the introduction necessarily asks what specific regulatory policy reforms might occur to provide a higher quality support worker labour force to improve client and public protection, as well as to enhance their often challenging work conditions in neo-liberal societies. It is clear that this needs to be based on an appropriate skill mix and interface with the health professions, as well as the hidden iceberg of unpaid informal carers who are just as invisible. As the chapters that make up this volume indicate, the answers may differ in the various societies considered, ranging from the introduction of tighter state-based regulation and support worker registers through placing greater requirements on employing organisations to developing more sensitive policies on migrant labour and the use of unpaid volunteers. Whatever policy solutions are offered, though, it is clear that the agenda is centrally pivoted on the management of risk to direct users, the wider public and support workers themselves in a fast-changing world with an increasingly ageing population.

In the latter respect, a major agenda going forward is that the voice of support workers themselves needs to be more fully heard, as highlighted by Baines and colleagues (2019). Although survey work among support workers is documented in several chapters of this volume, echoes of the voice of support workers are most strongly epitomised in the rich, qualitative interview with such a worker in Japan in Chapter eleven, which counterbalances the high level statistical analysis of personal support workers in Canada undertaken in Chapter ten. However, if we are going to fully grasp the predicaments in which support workers and their public find themselves in modern societies and move towards optimising their activities from the viewpoint of users and their carers, we need, among other things, to know more about how they experience the world – and how this impacts on their relationship with health professions, clients and other citizens. This is an area in which there is a comparative paucity of data, as underlined in Chapter five. Methodologically, applying more qualitative, quantitative and mixed methods in researching health (Saks and Allsop 2019) will help to fill the gap in moving forward the support worker field, which is so vital for all our futures. Central to this will be ensuring that there is appropriate health regulation in this area in the public interest (Chamberlain et al 2018).

As a postscript, the issue of the relationship of support workers, health professions and the public interest is accentuated by the recent global outbreak of COVID-19 that started in the first half of 2020. As has become ever more apparent, this has had huge implications for so many aspects of society. The self-isolation of members of the public has placed even more strain on support workers – both physically and mentally – especially in terms of the availability of unpaid informal carers. In a world of changing demographics, so too have the rising rates of morbidity and mortality from COVID-19 among the aged and other segments of the population in hospitals, care homes and the wider community. This highlights the need for well-regulated and managed support worker provision, working in harmony with professionalised members of the health and social care labour force, to protect their many clients. It also underlines that support workers themselves must be given appropriate protection for the sake of their own health and wellbeing in fulfilling their various roles on the frontline, alongside such key groups as doctors and nurses. Even more than ever before, in light of resource constraints in an economically challenged world, health support workers can no longer be regarded as marginal and invisible providers of health care.

Conclusion

In conclusion, it is worth reiterating the novelty of this edited book. While there are a number of articles on different aspects of support work in academic journals and other literature (see, for example, Williams et al 2015; Zeytinoglu et al 2014), there are, as previously noted, no equivalent social scientific books on this subject covering the areas concerned from a neo-Weberian perspective – still less including the interface of health support workers with the variety of health professions with whom they deal. Having said this, there are many practical books relating to support workers dealing with different aspects of their operation on the ground (see, for instance, Ebrahimi et al 2017; Peate 2017). These books, however, are largely training manuals for practitioners. As such, they do not offer substantive overlaps with this volume, as they at best only touch on the academic issues covered by this book. The volume also goes beyond research-based commissioned reports on health support work – such as those by Saks and colleagues (2000) and Cavendish (2013) in the UK; although based on research, they are typically written with a more focused policy purpose shaped by government agendas than this book, notwithstanding its own policy thrust.

This edited collection will be most warmly welcomed by the following groups: social scientific researchers in sociology, politics, policy, economics and related disciplines with interests in health support work and their relationship to the health professions; selected social science students on cognate courses at final year and postgraduate level; and higher level undergraduate and postgraduate students in the health professions. The book will also be very relevant to health support workers themselves, including those in the process of advanced training; the health professionals who increasingly oversee their work; and health care managers operating in relevant organisational contexts. This is in addition to the already indicated appeal to policy makers, including regulators – as well as an educated lay audience with interests in contemporary health issues. For those groups in higher education, this book may well be suitable reading on course programmes, as well as a reference guide for lecturers and researchers. To all the constituents to whom the book is directed, though, it is hoped that it brings sound academic thinking in driving forward an enhanced understanding of, and beneficial policy change in, health support work in the wider health care division of labour.

References

Baines, D., Kent, P. and Kent, S. (2019) ' "Off my own back": Precarity on the frontlines of care work', *Work, Employment and Society* 33(5): 877–87.

Borsay, A. and Hunter, B. (eds) (2012) *Nursing and Midwifery in Britain Since 1700*, Basingstoke: Palgrave Macmillan.

Cavendish, C. (2013) *An Independent Review into Healthcare Assistants and Support Workers in the NHS and Social Care Settings*, https://assets. publishing.service.gov.uk/government/uploads/system/uploads/ attachment_data/file/236212/Cavendish_Review.pdf

Chamberlain, J.M. (2015) *Medical Regulation, Fitness to Practise and Revalidation*, Bristol: Policy Press.

Chamberlain, J.M., Dent, M. and Saks, M. (eds) (2018) *Professional Health Regulation in the Public Interest: International Perspectives*, Bristol: Policy Press.

Dubois, C.-A., McKee, M. and Nolte, E. (eds) (2006) *Human Resources for Health in Europe*, Maidenhead: Open University Press.

Ebrahimi, V.A., Chapman, H.M. and Mann, T. (eds) (2017) *Reablement Services in Health and Social Care: A Guide to Practice for Students and Support Workers*, London: Palgrave.

Flood, J. (2018) 'Professions and professional service firms in a global context: Reframing narratives', in Saks, M. and Muzio, D. (eds) *Professions and Professional Service Firms: Private and Public Sector Enterprises in the Global Economy*, Abingdon: Routledge.

Larkin, G. (2002) 'Regulating the professions allied to medicine', in Allsop, J. and Saks, M. (eds) *Regulating the Health Professions*, London: Sage.

Lishman, J., Yuill, C., Brannan, J. and Gibson, A. (eds) (2018) *Social Work: An Introduction*, 2nd edition, London: Sage.

Nolan, F. (2003) *The Wild West: History, Myth and the Making of America*, Atlanta, GA: A Cappella.

Peate, I. (2017) *Fundamentals of Care: A Textbook for Health and Social Care Assistants*, Chichester: Wiley Blackwell.

Saks, M. (2010) 'Analyzing the professions: The case for a neo-Weberian approach', *Comparative Sociology* 9(6): 887–915.

Saks, M. (2015) 'Personal support workers: Learning from the UK in taming the Wild West', Keynote address, Ontario Community Support Association Conference, Toronto, Canada.

Saks, M. (2015) *The Professions, State and the Market: Medicine in Britain, the United States and Russia*, Abingdon: Routledge.

Saks, M. (2016a) 'Review of theories of professions, organizations and society: Neo-Weberianism, neo-institutionalism and eclecticism', *Journal of Professions and Organization* 3(2): 170–87.

Saks, M. (2016b) 'The regulation of the English health professions: Zoos, circuses or safari parks?', in Liljegren, A. and Saks, M. (eds) *Professions and Metaphors: Understanding Professions in Society*, Abingdon: Routledge.

Saks, M. and Allsop, J. (2007) 'Social policy, professional regulation and health support work in the United Kingdom', *Social Policy and Society* 6(2): 165–77.

Saks, M. and Allsop, J. (eds) (2019) *Researching Health: Qualitative, Quantitative and Mixed Methods*, 3rd edition, London: Sage.

Saks, M., Allsop, J., Chevannes, M., Clark, M., Fagan, R., Genders, N., Johnson, M., Kent, J., Payne, C., Price, D., Szczepura, A. and Unell, J. (2000) *Review of Health Support Workers*, Leicester: UK Departments of Health/De Montfort University.

Williams, A.P., Peckham, A., Kuluski, K., Lum, J., Warrick, N., Spalding, K., Tam, T., Bruce-Barrett, C., Grasic, M. and Im, J. (2015) 'Caring for care givers: Challenging the assumptions', *Healthcare Papers* 15(1): 62–66.

World Health Organization (2019) *Aging and Life Course*, www.who.int/ageing/en/

Zeytinoglu, I.U., Denton, M., Brookman, C. and Plenderleith, J. (2014) 'Task shifting policy in Ontario, Canada. Does it help personal support workers' intention to stay?', *Health Policy* 117(2): 176–89.

TWO

Health professionals, support workers and the precariat

Mike Saks and Katherine Zagrodney

Introduction

Following the theoretical themes of this book, this chapter primarily adopts a neo-Weberian approach to the analysis of health support workers. Health support workers are seen here, as throughout the volume, as paid frontline carers providing support to clients and their carers who are not qualified and registered as part of a profession (Manthorpe and Martineau 2008). The chapter starts by considering the notion of health professionalisation from a neo-Weberian viewpoint, which has brought with it considerable benefits for doctors and others based on a monopolistic position in the market in terms of income, status and power. More recently, though, there has been some debate about deprofessionalisation in a world in which the rewards of professions are often seen to have been diminished by various changing socio-political circumstances. For neo-Marxists this equates to proletarianisation linked to the labour process in capitalist development which is in turn related to membership of the precariat (Han 2018). In this sense, both of these perspectives have a bearing on the relative positioning of health support workers and their precarity or otherwise. They therefore merit initial consideration as they threaten to muddy the water in understanding the socioeconomic situation of this occupational group.

Health support workers by definition do not fit the neo-Weberian notion of professions, but they are groups, as will be seen, whose conditions of work can very often be described as immiserated, even in comparison with those occupations at the bottom of the health professional pecking order and in relation to the proletariat in classic Marxist writing. It is on such health support workers that this chapter focuses – critically considering whether they can be seen as members of the precariat, which neo-Marxists sometimes believe has replaced the proletariat in terms of system-changing class consciousness within capitalism, or simply exist in a comparatively precarious position in the market from a neo-Weberian perspective. This discussion particularly centres on the comparative cases of Canada and the UK – in the latter case focused largely on England given the variations in each of the UK's four countries resulting from their increasingly devolved political authority. The chapter concludes by examining the policy implications of the analysis from the viewpoint of the theoretical concept of precarity.

Health professionalisation, deprofessionalisation and proletarianisation

The starting point, though, is neo-Weberianism, which sees health professions such as medicine, nursing and midwifery as based on exclusionary social closure in an ever-shifting marketplace (Saks 2010). Health professions in this framework in the Anglo-American context have typically gained legal monopolies underwritten by the state, centred on restrictive registers excluding outsiders. This enables greater socioeconomic rewards to be gained by such middle and upper class groups in the market, in contrast to most of those who are excluded. The main power base of excluded groups tends to be centred on unions and industrial action of the traditional working class in a position of usurpationary closure. Indeed, some professions themselves like nursing can be viewed as combining elements of both types of closure – giving rise to the term 'dual closure' (Parkin 1979). More recently, parallel tensions have been represented as 'hybridisation', whereby organisational and professional logics come into conflict and are mediated by professional groups in interstitial roles (Noordegraaf 2018), as empirically depicted in nursing by Carvalho (2014). Health support workers – on which this chapter and the book is centred – are those that have yet to professionalise and therefore can be seen to be part of the excluded cluster of occupational groups, while still carrying out one or more of the many diverse forms of caring for users of services in modern societies (Saks and Allsop 2007).

It is in this context that arguments have been put, on both sides of the Atlantic, that a process of deprofessionalisation is generally occurring in the professions – not so much in terms of eroding the exclusionary social closure of professions, whether through state-by-state licensing or statutory regulation at national level, as by reducing their associated rewards (Saks 2016a). This has been held to have taken place in both public and private sector settings, particularly as professions and expert professional knowledge have come under increasing neo-liberal challenge with a growing emphasis on market efficiency and the sovereignty of the consumer. According to contributors like Dent and colleagues (2004) and Flood (2018), this move has been associated with the rise of the New Public Management which has led, among other things, to the rise of disaggregation, competition and incentivisation undermining the elevated position of professions even in non-privatised settings, although this has to some degree been counterbalanced by their resistance and adaptability. In this respect, aside from the deployment of professional power and interests, the development of such future roles of professions as risk managers in a risk society and trusted interpreters of information may help in protecting and even advancing their standing (Leicht 2018).

In the classically dominant position of medicine itself, at the pinnacle of the professional hierarchy, there has been much debate about deprofessionalisation. As Saks (2015) notes, there is no necessary convergence in this trend between societies, not least given historical and contemporary socio-political variations in the relationship between professions, state and the market. Thus, in North America in the more market-oriented case of the United States there is evidence of a decline in income, status and power among less prestigious specialisms in face of rising corporatisation that has driven down both costs and clinical autonomy. In the UK, though, the state medical shelter of the NHS has ensured that there has not been a significant decline in the overall professional standing of doctors, but rather restratification between general practitioners and consultants with the growing influence of the former over decision making at national and local level – despite the recent establishment of more regulatory oversight of medical self-regulation (Chamberlain 2015). Meanwhile in Canada, the comparative case considered here in relation to health support workers, physicians have continued to rule the roost in a society with less focus on primary care (Hutchinson et al 2011), retaining to a great degree their self-regulatory powers (Ahmed et al 2018).

Neo-Marxists, however, dress this up by redefining some of the more erosive processes at work as proletarianisation rather than deprofessionalisation. This is linked to the inexorable dynamics of the development of capitalism in which some mid- and high-ranking positions are reduced to that of the proletariat in the labour process. This is well exemplified by Braverman (1998), who believed that the roles of health professional groups like nurses were being broken down as a result of increasing managerial efforts, through Taylorism and beyond, to control the labour process and decrease wage costs. Such views about the inevitability of proletarianisation have also been manifested in medicine by neo-Marxist writers like McKinlay and Arches (1985), although Navarro (1986) clouds the issue by seeing doctors as part of the capitalist class itself, even if they do not in themselves own the means of production. Either way this politicised neo-Marxist view of proletarianisation, in which capitalist society is held to be inexorably polarising on class lines, departs from that of neo-Weberians who tend to focus on such issues as increased bureaucratisation, competition from other occupational groups and the growth of consumer power in the market in accounting for any trends to deprofessionalisation (see, for instance, Haug 1988).

In assessing these trends empirically, whether they are seen as deprofessionalisation or proletarianisation or some other end state, it is important to recognise that this is a complex task and there are a number of methodological bear traps. These include the choice of indicators that might be most helpful in gauging the extent of deprofessionalisation/professionalisation or the further proletarianisation/embourgoisement of the health professional labour force. In the case of doctors, Elston (1991) highlights various aspects of the range of benchmarking criteria that could be employed from the control of medical education and training, levels of remuneration and the degree of lay influence over medicine to the skilling of medical tasks, non-medical encroachment and the unionisation of doctors. There are also comparative international methodological issues to be addressed where more than one society is involved (Burau 2019), questions about the timescale to be employed and why this has been chosen in judging the claims being made (Light 1995). This complexity underlines the methodological difficulties involved in looking at other facets of the dynamic health care division of labour, which – as will be seen – includes the extent to which health support workers can be viewed as part of the new precariat.

Health support workers and the concept of the precariat

In this sense, it is clear that – whatever the socioeconomic position of doctors and other health professionals in the neo-liberal societies of the UK and Canada in response to developments such as growing corporatisation, more active citizen lobbies and greater state engagement – the support workers who engage with them still largely exist in a more emaciated condition. The evidence for this is set out in the next sections of the chapter, but it is first necessary to introduce the key concept of precarity, around which the discussion is focused. The origins of this concept are definitely neo-Marxist, of which Standing (2011) has been the key advocate. He argues that a new class called the precariat has arisen in neo-liberal societies with increasing privatisation of the welfare state and the spread of the New Public Management. It includes many lowly paid people, often of female gender and ethnic origin, leading insecure work lives characterised by short-term contracts, who have the potential to develop a collective class consciousness. As such, the precariat is seen to represent a new force for revolutionary change in a situation of unstable and unpredictable working conditions. This contrasts with the classic Marxist conception of the proletariat, although both share a lack of ownership of the means of production and are clearly linked. However, the proletariat is viewed as having more security in the labour market, especially given such developments as the growing legal responsibilities of employers, improved occupational health and safety, enhanced workplace representation, stronger income streams and greater opportunities for upward social mobility. As we shall highlight in this chapter, the precariat lacks much of that security, stability and predictability.

However, the neo-Marxist notion of the precariat does not mean that the analysis of precarity lacks a neo-Weberian base. The concept of precarious employment has existed in parallel for a number of years based on such features as low wages and job insecurity (see, for instance, Vosko 2006). It is perfectly *de rigueur* for neo-Weberians to highlight such consequences of the operation of the market in modern neo-liberal societies. What it is not so readily possible to accept is the deterministic statements of neo-Marxists about the developing class consciousness of this newly identified precariat – following in the footsteps of earlier judgements in the 19th and 20th centuries about the inexorable rise of the proletariat, resulting in political activity leading to the overthrow of capitalism and the establishment of socialism (Blackledge 2011). Part of this evaluation of the concept of the precariat in relation to health support work will therefore explore the likelihood of it spawning the common consciousness now envisaged, as well as examining in the illustrative context of the UK and Canada whether the work of health support workers is indeed precarious (Johnson 2015) – a crucial aspect that has all too infrequently been empirically examined, with the exception of such generic work as that in the UK by Savage and colleagues (2013) and the more specific reviews by contributors like Zagrodney and Saks (2017) in Canada.

This is a vital area given that health support workers conduct such a wide range of roles from health care aides to nursing assistants, forming the greatest part of the health workforce in the UK and other neo-liberal societies (see, for instance, Saks and Allsop 2007). As such, they fill the gap between informal and professionally-instigated care in domiciliary and institutional settings, often bringing together for the end user silo-based professional delivery in an age where a growing proportion of the population is ageing and experiencing multiple chronic conditions (United Nations Population Fund 2012). There is existing evidence too that in countries spanning from Australia and Denmark to France and The Netherlands health support workers are more likely to be older women and of minority extraction (Fujisawa and Colombo 2009), who are frequently faced with low wages and job insecurity (Korczyk 2004). Furthermore, a recent international study by Jokela (2019) found that domestic workers have a higher probability of working in precarious employment settings in five societies with welfare states, as compared to other industries. This general picture of precarity is also endorsed by Polson (2013) in the United States who charts the growth of a low-waged sporadically politicised health support worker labour force operating in places like New York City between the formal and informal economy. Progress on behalf of its mainly female and ethnic workforce has been made with union support in the push for living wages. However, multiple dimensions of precariousness are seen to remain, with particular vulnerability in recessionary conditions to issues like labour market insecurity and control of the labour process.

So what then of the illustrative case studies of the UK and Canada? How far do these cases sustain or otherwise the notion of precarity and the precariat in the context of the preceding paragraphs? The two countries have been chosen for comparison in part following guidance by Burau (2019) who suggests that – depending on the research purpose – it can be helpful to compare countries where there are strong selective similarities. In this instance, although geographically thousands of miles apart, both the UK and Canada share a common political heritage, and have similar forms of stable liberal democratic government and parallel passions for equitable and effective health care delivery – even if there are differences in such aspects as the balance of public and private health care, lay engagement in health care, the level of devolved professional regulatory authority and the independence of the medical profession (see Deber and Mah 2014; Saks 2015). There were pragmatic factors underpinning the choice too, including the UK and Canadian base of the authors and their mutual interest in studying their respective health systems – not least in relation to health support workers who are referred to in Canada as personal support workers

(PSWs). The UK is analysed first in examining the applicability of the concept of the precariat.

Health support workers and the precariat in the UK

The international characteristics of the precariat in modern societies on both sides of the Atlantic have certainly been mirrored in good measure in the UK. Here Saks and colleagues (2000) conducted what was the first, and still remains the most thorough, review of health support workers commissioned by the UK Departments of Health. This study found that this workforce numbered well over 1 million people, with many fluid cross-over points between health and social care, not least in Northern Ireland which has more formally integrated provision. Although the review was focused on risk and risk mitigation, it was clear from the analysis that such workers were generally not as strongly positioned in the market as they might be from the viewpoint of vocationally-based training and formal qualifications. There were some notable exceptions to this, like operating department practitioners who have now professionalised in a neo-Weberian sense, but in overall terms such support workers were sufficiently poorly paid to question whether they could even contribute low-grade fees to support a minimal mandatory register – distinct from a full professional register – to protect the public. If such a register was instigated, this was seen as of necessity largely a government responsibility, with a relatively low contribution to the costs by the staff themselves.

This picture, which points to the precarity of many health support workers in the UK, is reinforced by the more recent review by Cavendish (2013) which refers to the 1.3 million frontline health and care staff who deliver most of the hands-on care in hospitals, care homes and the homes of individuals – of which 84 per cent are female, with 15 per cent in health care and 29 per cent in social care drawn from black and minority ethnic groups. The review highlighted the deficiencies in the current position of such support workers by, among other things, recommending greater educational certification and career opportunities for support workers. From the viewpoint of precarity, it also proposed the payment of travel expenses to those on zero-hours contracts since otherwise earnings may fall below the national minimum wage. Having said this, the review did note the variation in pay bands in the NHS and the lower pay in the private sector. Moreover, workers in social care environments such as residential homes for the elderly were not only substantially more poorly paid than professional social workers, but also typically had a lower income than support workers in the health sector – in which pay and status are not exactly high. In part because of this, the very loose link between pay and performance, and the high stress and sickness rates related to the frequent long shift pattern for support workers, there were relatively large rates of attrition among support workers in health and social care.

These precarious job characteristics were also found in other studies of this much neglected group of workers that have for long been at the margins of official health care (Saks 2008). Support workers remain marginal in the most recent reports which focus on the 1.5 million strong health professional workforce. This is despite the growing importance and utilisation of support workers in part as a response to an increase in the elderly population and long-term conditions and the strains that this imposes on the professionally qualified deliverers of health care (see, for example, Public Health England 2017). Nonetheless, several other publications testify to the difficult employment conditions that health support workers continue to experience. In an early study Thornley (1997), for instance, highlighted such issues in relation to the invisible work of health care assistants in the NHS. More recently Dyer and colleagues (2008) underlined that care work is typically low paid in the UK and is undertaken in precarious, informal, or temporary situations. They also documented that many of these largely female populated posts are filled by economic migrants – a point which is reinforced by McDowell and colleagues (2009) in the context of Greater London service work more generally. Barron and West (2013), meanwhile, discovered in their large-scale study that, as in North America, there was a statistically significant wage penalty in the UK for working in occupations involved in providing care for others, especially for those like nursing assistants and auxiliaries with lower level qualifications. Overall, such available literature suggests many precarious features of support workers in the UK.

Accepting the precarity of many of these health support workers does not necessarily mean that they will coalesce in a neo-Marxist sense in future to form a fully self-aware class of similarly placed employees aimed at the overthrow of capitalism. To be sure, there have been minority political movements in the UK, as symbolised by the Democracy Village established in 2010 in Parliament Square outside Westminster, which have been anti-capitalist. Unions, like Unison which represents the public services, have also been very aware of the plight of a large number of health support workers and have fought their cause on a longstanding basis (see, for example, Thornley 1998). But, given that such workers have more than 300 job titles (Saks and Allsop 2007), most of which lack clear job descriptions and competencies, are inconsistently used, and are associated with enormous variation in the tasks undertaken at different rates of pay (Cavendish 2013), the chances of a radical self-identifying precariat class emerging seem slim. The ability for such a diverse as well as a physically divided group of workers to act as a single entity may be too ambitious an expectation at present. This is particularly so when it is appreciated that their roles span from unqualified workers within clinical and therapeutic teams and independent practitioners within as yet emerging professions to those providing face-to-face care in clients' own homes and work in private and public sector institutional contexts (Saks 2008). What, though, of the parallel case of PSWs and the precariat in Canada?

Personal support workers and the precariat in Canada

The position of PSWs in the labour market of the neo-liberal health care system of Canada is not vastly different from the UK. However, the Canadian literature is either largely focused on provinces and territories rather than at the federal level or national in scope, but restricted to given sectors where PSWs operate such as the home care sector. The interest in differences by care sector follows from the scenario in Canada, where health care has also increasingly moved from hospitals and more general institutional care to the home and community (Health Council of Canada 2012). With a consequent growing dependence on home care, some 30,000 PSWs were found to be working in this sector alone nationally in an early study by the Home Care Sector Corporation (2003). Moreover, the overall numbers of PSWs in Ontario, the largest province, has been estimated at around 100,000 (Health Professions Regulatory Advisory Council 2006), which gives some indication of the scale of this workforce across the ten provinces and three territories of Canada. This may in total number close to 1 million – with ever growing demand (see, for example, Bloom et al 2012). As in the UK, moreover, staff in this sector are mainly older and female – with a higher proportion of visible minority and ethnic status relative to the general employed population (Lum et al 2010). There is also a lack of mandatory educational training programmes across Canada, although a variable patchwork of requirements for these exists in health care in different provinces, regions, sectors and employments. This contributes to the largely depressed status of PSWs but is not the whole story as to why many have low esteem and market value (Kelly 2017).

Although there are variations in such areas as financial rewards for PSWs across the provinces and territories of Canada (Church et al

2004), similarities between PSWs and the archetypical precariat also abound in terms of the nature of their work. For example, Canadian PSWs like UK health support workers seem regularly to transfer backwards and forwards into other parallel work roles and their pay is mostly very low (see, for example, Zeytinoglu et al 2009). Earnings in fact are typically around or below a living wage, with the most limited rates in home and community care (Lilly 2008), in which registered nurses earn approximately double that of PSWs on average (Home Care Sector Study Corporation 2003). In addition, PSWs in Canada are largely engaged in part-time roles, with casual hours and short-term contracts (see, among others, Zeytinoglu et al 2014). Although the majority of Canadian PSWs often report union status, the degree of unionisation varies greatly by employment characteristics and geographic location – including by province (Sims-Gould et al 2010). Involvement with a union, while inconsistent, can help to protect pay and job security as well as enhance wages. However, the positive effects of union status is counteracted by the identified low upward social mobility of this group of workers and the large amount of unpaid labour their work usually involves (Nugent 2007). Migrant status also substantially and negatively impacts the precarious nature of this field (Goldring and Landolt 2013).

On this basis, it appears that a large number of PSWs, like health support workers in the UK, can be identified as operating in conditions of precarity in both neo-Weberian and neo-Marxist terms. Caution, though, again needs to be made about making blanket statements about all PSWs being members of the precariat in this sense, given the variations in the range of workplace characteristics that exist in different locations and sectors of the market. It should not be forgotten that some support worker roles, as in the UK, are stable, full-time and quite well paid in relation to the tasks performed. Nonetheless, most of this workforce can be seen as part of the precariat and evidence from Canada suggests that that the predominant features of PSW labour like part-time working, casual hours, job insecurity and heavy workloads with too little support result in high degrees of stress and low job satisfaction (Denton et al 2002). There also seems to be a relationship with physical as well as mental health (Zeytinoglu et al 2015), with musculoskeletal injuries being the most reported issue (Ngan et al 2010). The precarious conditions of PSWs linked to the high risk of mental or physical sickness at work also mean that staff turnover and absence are quite high – which has negative consequences for users and employers in terms of continuity of care (Zeytinoglu et al 2009).

However, as in the UK, there are good reasons for holding back on assuming that – in accord with the neo-Marxist vision – such precarity will inevitably lead to the emergence of a class-conscious group of PSWs with the development of advanced capitalism. Despite anger sporadically being expressed through unions about their working conditions (Chun 2016a) and documented successes in working with these unions (Vosko 2006), PSWs and the workforce more generally in Canada do not appear to currently be particularly politically conscious, with comparatively limited affiliation with politicised associations representing PSWs. Indeed, membership of collective groups such as unions or cognate associations (for instance, Ontario Personal Support Workers Association) is inconsistent – with only up to a fifth of this occupational group at present being members of unions in Canada, despite the political impetus and the tangible benefits that such membership can bring (Hewko et al 2015). The future direction as regards a potential political movement based on PSWs also appears limited given their parallel differentiation by role and sector to that in the UK, which seems likely to impede the development of their collective identity and consciousness as a class (Zagrodney and Saks 2017). This accentuates the great heterogeneity of the Canadian PSW labour force, which is further explored in Chapter ten of this volume. The policy implications of the position of health support workers as members of a putative precariat in the UK, Canada and beyond are now considered in the conclusion.

Conclusion: health support workers, precarity and future policy

The precarity of the health support worker labour force in the UK and Canada therefore appears similar in both countries. This is highlighted by the cross-national comparative qualitative study in Scotland and Canada by Cunningham and colleagues (2016) on the conditions and experience of employment in two non-profit social service agencies. This precarity is especially accentuated relative to the health professions in general and medicine in particular – notwithstanding any potential deprofessionalisation or proletarianisation to which they may be subject. As such, the application of the concept of precarity therefore is compatible in principle with a neo-Weberian and a neo-Marxist theoretical approach – linked to the dynamics of the market or production respectively – despite the frailties both sometimes evince in their operationalisation (Saks 2016b). However, as Muntaner (2016) notes, the concept of precarious work is still open to a number of challenges. Such challenges include: how far precarious employment, as frequently implied, is a new phenomenon in health support work and other areas; to what degree precarious employment can be said to be generalised across countries; and the extent to which it is simply a manifestation of working class employment rather than a separate entity to be analysed in itself.

A further challenge of central interest to us here concerns the political destination of those engaged in precarious employment, particularly from a neo-Marxist viewpoint. Where this is moving in the future in terms of class consciousness is a moot point. It seems unlikely that a revolutionary consciousness will develop simply from the seeds of their relative deprivation, given the fragmentation of this section of the labour force – including, as has been seen, among health support workers themselves both geographically, even within a single nation, and in terms of membership of unions. Classic theorists of revolution like Davies (1971) highlight that it is too simplistic to think that deprivation in relation to other groups itself causes revolution, otherwise the masses would always be in revolt. This said, globally there have been signs of recent resistance by the working poor and socially marginalised against austerity through various anti-capitalist political movements such as the Occupy movement in London in the UK, as mirrored in the United States. Yet there are serious doubts as to whether their frustration can translate into sustained activism and class solidarity in the longer run, transforming a 'class-in-itself' into a 'class-for-itself' in the neo-Marxist idiom, not least in relation to health support workers and employees in kindred occupations (Chun 2016b).

However, from a policy viewpoint it is certainly appropriate to consider whether groups like health care assistants will take a high or low road in the future (Thornley 2003). There may indeed be an imperative for neo-liberal governments to ameliorate the situation of support workers, if only to help ensure an adequate supply of such workers on the labour market by improving recruitment and retention to meet rising demand on a global stage. Indeed, in liberal democratic societies with egalitarian and social welfare policies like the UK and Canada, human rights may also be a driver to enhance the position of health support workers. Standing (2011) certainly sees such rights as very limited for the wider precariat in terms of their civil, cultural, social, economic and political dimensions. Drawing mainly on examples from the UK, Mantouvalou (2012) in fact argues that legislative precariousness may be created because of the special vulnerability created by the exclusion or lower extent of protection of certain categories of these workers from protective laws, as in the case of domestic work. Nonetheless, Standing (2014) has proposed solutions to precarity in a recent book entitled *A Precarity Charter*, in which he warns of the dangers of capture by right-wing extremists. His hope is that the middle and upper classes, including the professions, will foster a new top-down progressive politics in neo-liberal societies supporting social justice for health support workers and other members of the precariat.

While this may give too little credit to the capacity of short-run bottom-up endeavours to effect socio-political change (Chun 2016b), some governments and public and private sector institutions have already endeavoured to act further to address the multifactorial malaise of precarity afflicting health support workers. Thus in Ontario, for example, the Ministry has put in place measures to mitigate the risk to public health and safety by addressing market deficiencies on the supply side – including systemic wage increases and rising investment in PSW training – while task shifting has been proposed for service providers to make support worker roles more engaging (Zeytinoglu et al 2014). Although there may still be a misalignment between precarious labour and regulatory laws and employment norms in Canada (Zhang and Zuberi 2017), in the UK there has been less proactivity, with some changes such as the reform of the Overseas Domestic Workers (ODW) visa regime representing a backward step (Mullally 2015). However, with ever growing health care costs and the omnipresent knock on effects of Brexit for the European health care labour supply, it may only be a question of time before a stronger appreciation of the value of health support workers takes root. Societies like the UK may pride themselves on their comparatively high employment rates, but the nature of that employment is vital. When so much of the health care labour market involves socially excluded health support workers in precarious jobs, with features such as short-term contracts, low wages and insecurity, the time for greater and more focused policy reform has surely been reached.

References

Ahmed, H., Brown, A. and Saks, M. (2018) 'Patterns of medical oversight and regulation in Canada', in Chamberlain, J.M., Dent, M. and Saks, M. (eds) *Professional Health Regulation in the Public Interest: International Perspectives*, Bristol: Policy Press.

Barron, D.N. and West, E. (2013) 'The financial costs of caring in the British labour market: Is there a wage penalty for workers in caring occupations?', *British Journal of Industrial Relations* 51(1): 104–23.

Blackledge, P. (2011) *Reflections on the Marxist Theory of History*, Manchester: Manchester University Press.

Bloom, J., Duckett, S. and Robertson, A. (2012) 'Development of an interactive model for planning the care workforce for Alberta: Case study', *Human Resources for Health* 10: 22.

Braverman, H. (1998) *Labor and Monopoly Capital: The Degradation of Work in the Twentieth Century*, New edition, New York: Monthly Review Press.

Burau, V. (2019) 'Comparative health research', in Saks, M. and Allsop, J. (eds) *Researching Health: Qualitative, Quantitative and Mixed Methods*, 3rd edition, London: Sage.

Carvahlo, T. (2014) 'Changing connections between professionalism and managerialism: A case study of nursing in Portugal', *Journal of Professions and Organization* 1(2): 176–90.

Cavendish, C. (2013) *An Independent Review into Healthcare Assistants and Support Workers in the NHS and Social Care Settings*, https://assets.publishing.service.gov.uk/government/uploads/system/uploads/attachment_data/file/236212/Cavendish_Review.pdf

Chamberlain, J.M. (2015) *Medical Regulation, Fitness to Practise and Revalidation*, Bristol: Policy Press.

Chun, J.J. (2016a) 'Organizing across divides: Union challenges to precarious work in Vancouver's privatized health care sector', *Progress in Development Studies* 16(2): 173–88.

Chun, J.J. (2016b) 'The affective politics of the precariat: Reconsidering alternative histories of grassroots worker organising', *Global Labour Journal* 7(2): 136–47.

Church, K., Diamond, T. and Voronka, J. (2004) *In Profile: Personal Support Workers in Canada*, Toronto: RBC Institute for Disability Studies Research and Education, Ryerson University.

Cunningham, I., Baines, D., Shields, J. and Lewchuk, W. (2016) 'Austerity policies, "precarity" and the nonprofit workforce: A comparative study of UK and Canada', *Journal of Industrial Relations* 58(4): 455–72.

Davies, J.C. (ed) (1971) *When Men Revolt and Why: A Reader in Political Violence and Revolution*, New York: Free Press.

Deber, R.B. and Mah, C.L. (eds) (2014) *Case Studies in Canadian Health Policy and Management*, Toronto: Toronto University Press.

Dent, M., Chandler, J. and Barry, J. (eds) (2004) *Questioning the New Public Management*, Aldershot: Ashgate.

Denton, M., Zeytinoglu, I.U., Davies, S. and Lian, J. (2002) 'Job stress and job dissatisfaction of home care workers in the context of health care restructuring', *International Journal of Health Services* 32(2): 327–57.

Dyer, S., McDowell, L. and Batnitzky, A. (2008) 'Emotional labour/body work: The caring labours of migrants in the UK's National Health Service', *Geoforum* 39(6): 2030–38.

Elston, M.A. (1991) 'The politics of professional power: Medicine in a changing health service', in Gabe, J., Calnan, M. and Bury, M. (eds) *The Sociology of the Health Service*, London: Routledge.

Flood, J. (2018) 'Professions and professional service firms in a global context: Reframing narratives', in Saks, M. and Muzio, D. (eds) *Professions and Professional Service Firms: Private and Public Sector Enterprises in the Global Economy*, Abingdon: Routledge.

Fujisawa, R. and Colombo, F. (2009) *The Long-term Care Workforce: Overview and Strategies to Adapt Supply to a Growing Demand. OECD Health Working Papers No. 44*, Paris: OECD.

Goldring, L. and Landolt, P. (2013) 'Caught in the work–citizenship matrix: The lasting effects of precarious legal status on work for Toronto immigrants', in Munk, R., Schierup, C.U. and Wise, R.D. (eds) *Migration, Work and Citizenship in the New Global Order*, Abingdon: Routledge.

Han, C. (2018) 'Precarity, precariousness, and vulnerability', *Annual Review of Anthropology* 47: 331–43.

Haug, M. (1988) 'A re-examination of the hypothesis of physician deprofessionalization', *Milbank Quarterly* 66: 48–56.

Health Council of Canada (2012) *Seniors in Need, Caregivers in Distress: What Are the Home Care Priorities for Seniors?* Ottawa: HCC.

Health Professions Regulatory Advisory Council (2006) 'The regulation of personal support workers', *Health Professions Regulatory Advisory Council*, Toronto: HPRAC.

Hewko, S.J., Cooper, S.L., Huynh, H., Spiwek, T.L., Carleton, H.L., Reid, S. and Cummings, G.G. (2015) 'Invisible no more: A scoping review of the health care aide workforce literature', *BMC Nursing* 14(38).

Home Care Sector Study Corporation (2003) *Canadian Home Care Human Resources Study*, Ottawa: Canadian Research Network for Care in the Community.

Hutchinson, B., Levesque, J.F., Strumpf, E. and Coyle, N. (2011) 'Primary health care in Canada: Systems in motion', *Milbank Quarterly* 89(2): 256–88.

Johnson, M. (ed) (2015) *Precariat: Labour, Work and Politics*, Abingdon: Routledge.

Jokela, M. (2019) 'Patterns of precarious employment in a female-dominated sector in five welfare states – The case of paid domestic labor sector', *Social Politics* 26(1).

Kelly, C. (2017) 'Exploring experiences of Personal Support Worker education in Ontario, Canada', *Health and Social Care in the Community*, https://doi:10.1111/hsc.12443.

Korczyk, S.M. (2004) *Long-term Workers in Five Countries: Issues and Options*, Washington DC: Public Policy Institute AARP.

Leicht, K. (2018) 'Professions and entrepreneurship in international perspective', in Saks, M. and Muzio, D. (eds) *Professions and Professional Service Firms: Private and Public Sector Enterprises in the Global Economy*, Abingdon: Routledge.

Light, D. (1995) 'Countervailing powers: A framework for professions in transition', in Johnson, T., Larkin, G. and Saks, M. (eds) *Health Professions and the State in Europe*, London: Routledge.

Lilly, M.B. (2008) 'Medical versus social work-places: Constructing and compensating the personal support worker across health care settings in Ontario, Canada', *Gender, Place and Culture* 15(3): 285–99.

Lum, J., Sladek, J. and Ying, A. (2010) 'Ontario personal support workers in home and community care: CRNCC/PSNO survey results', Ottawa: Canadian Research Network for Care in the Community.

McDowell, L., Batnitzky, A. and Dyer, S. (2009) 'Precarious work and economic migration: Emerging immigrant divisions of labour in Greater London's service sector', *International Journal of Urban and Regional Research* 33(1): 3–25.

McKinlay, J. and Arches, J. (1985) 'Towards the proletarianization of physicians', *International Journal of Health Services* 18: 161–95.

Manthorpe, J. and Martineau, S. (2008) *Support Workers: Their Role and Tasks: A Scoping Review*, London: King's College.

Mantouvalou, V. (2012) 'Human rights for precarious workers: The legislative precariousness of domestic labor', *Comparative Labor Law and Policy Journal* 34(1).

Mullally, S. (2015) 'Migrant domestic workers in the UK: Enacting exclusions, exemptions and rights', in Mullally, S. (ed) *Care, Migration and Human Rights: Law and Practice*, Abingdon: Routledge.

Muntaner, C. (2016) 'Global precarious employment and health inequalities: Working conditions, social class, or precariat?', *Cadernos de saude publica 32*.

Navarro, V. (1986) *Crisis, Health and Medicine: A Social Critique*, London: Tavistock.

Noordegraaf, M. (2018) 'Enterprise, hybrid professionalism and the public sector', in Saks, M. and Muzio, D. (eds) *Professions and Professional Service Firms: Private and Public Sector Enterprises in the Global Economy*. Abingdon: Routledge.

Ngan K., Drebit, S., Siow, S., Yu, S., Keen, D. and Alamgir, H. (2010) 'Risks and causes of musculoskeletal injuries among health care workers', *Occupational Medicine* 60(5): 389–94.

Nugent, L.S. (2007) 'Can't they get anything better? Home support workers call for change', *Home Health Care Services Quarterly* 26(2): 21–39.

Parkin, F. (1979) *Marxism and Class Theory: A Bourgeois Critique*, London: Tavistock.

Polson, D. (2013) 'The caring precariat: home health care work in New York City', PhD thesis, City University of New York.

Public Health England (2017) *Facing the Facts, Shaping the Future: A Draft Health and Care Workforce Strategy for England to 2027*, London: Health Education England.

Saks, M. (2008) 'Policy dynamics: Marginal groups in the healthcare division of labour in the UK', in Kuhlmann, E. and Saks, M. (eds) *Rethinking Professional Governance: International Directions in Healthcare*, Bristol: Policy Press.

Saks, M. (2010) 'Analyzing the professions: The case for a neo-Weberian approach', *Comparative Sociology* 9(6): 887–915.

Saks, M. (2015) *The Professions, State and the Market: Medicine in Britain, the United States and Russia*, Abingdon: Routledge.

Saks, M. (2016a) 'Professions and power', in Dent, M., Bourgeault, I., Dennis, J. and Kuhlmann, E. (eds) *The Routledge Companion to the Professions and Professionalism*, Abingdon: Routledge.

Saks, M. (2016b) 'Review of theories of professions, organizations and society: Neo-Weberianism, neo-institutionalism and eclecticism', *Journal of Professions and Organization* 3(2): 170–87.

Saks, M. and Allsop, J. (2007) 'Social policy, professional regulation and health support work in the United Kingdom', *Social Policy and Society* 6(2): 165–77.

Saks, M., Allsop, J., Chevannes, M., Clark, M., Fagan, R., Genders, N., Johnson, M., Kent, J., Payne, C., Price, D., Szczepura, A. and Unell, J. (2000) *Review of Health Support Workers. Report to the UK Departments of Health*, Leicester: UK Departments of Health/De Montfort University.

Savage, M., Devine, F., Cunningham, N., Taylor, M., Li, Y., Hjellbrekke, J., Le Roux, B., Friedman, S. and Miles, A. (2013) 'A new model of social class? Findings from the BBC's Great British Class Survey Experiment', *Sociology* 47(2): 219–50.

Sims-Gould, J., Byrne, K., Craven, C., Martin-Matthews, A. and Keefe, J. (2010) 'Why I became a home support worker: Recruitment in the home health sector', *Home Health Care Services Quarterly* 29(4):171–94.

Standing, G. (2011) *The Precariat: The New Dangerous Class*, London: Bloomsbury Academic.

Standing, G. (2014) *A Precariat Charter: From Denizens to Citizens*, London: Bloomsbury Academic.

Thornley, C. (1997) *The Invisible Workers: An Investigation into the Pay and Employment of Health Care Assistants in the NHS*, London: Unison.

Thornley, C. (1998) *Neglected Nurses, Hidden Work: An Investigation into the Pay and Employment of Nursing Auxiliaries/Assistants in the NHS*, London: Unison.

Thornley, C. (2003) 'What future for health care assistants: High road or low road?', in Davies, C. (ed) *The Future Health Workforce*, Basingstoke: Palgrave.

United Nations Population Fund (2012) *Ageing in the Twenty-First Century: A Celebration and a Challenge*, New York: UNPF.

Vosko, L.F. (ed) (2006) *Precarious Employment: Understanding Labour Market Insecurity in Canada*, Montreal: McGill-Queen's University Press.

Zagrodney, K. and Saks, M. (2017) 'Personal support workers in Canada: The new precariat?', *Healthcare Policy* 13(2): 31–9.

Zeytinoglu, I.U., Denton, M., Davies, S. and Plenderleith, J. (2009) 'Casualized employment and turnover intention: Home care workers in Ontario, Canada', *Health Policy* 91(3): 258–68.

Zeytinoglu, I.U., Denton, M., Brookman, C. and Plenderleith, J. (2014) 'Task shifting policy in Ontario, Canada. Does it help personal support workers' intention to stay?', *Health Policy* 117(2): 176–89.

Zeytinoglu, I.U., Denton, M., Plenderleith, J. and Chowhan, J. (2015) 'Associations between workers' health, and non-standard hours and insecurity: The case of home care workers in Ontario, Canada', *International Journal of Human Resource Management* 26(19): 2503–22.

Zhang, S. and Zuberi, D. (2017) 'Evening the keel: Measuring and responding to precarity in the Canadian labour economy', *Canadian Public Administration* 60(1): 28–47.

THREE

Unpaid informal carers: The 'shadow' workforce in health care

A. Paul Williams and Janet M. Lum

Introduction

As Starr (1982) has observed, the 20th century marked the rise of scientific medicine and a shift in the site of care from people's homes to hospitals, which he characterised as 'citadels of science'. While previously most people were born and died at home, now they are born and die in the hospital. The 21st century marks the reversal of that trend. As illnesses that can be cured on an episodic basis in hospitals are supplanted by multiple chronic health and social needs that cannot be cured, and must be managed over the long term, the big policy push across industrialised countries is to shift more care to community settings. Justifications include that, in ageing societies, growing numbers of older persons with ongoing care needs wish to 'age at home'; hospital visits are costly; and lengthy hospital stays, particularly for frail older persons, can pose serious risks of hospital-borne illnesses and a progressive loss of functional capacity due to inactivity and lack of restorative care.

This shift in the site of care also fundamentally changes the line-up of people who provide care. In hospitals, well paid, highly trained, highly regulated and highly visible professionals such as doctors, nurses, technologists and therapists deliver or direct most care. Beyond the hospital walls, these professionals – based on exclusionary social closure from a neo-Weberian perspective (Saks 2010) – have a more limited presence. Instead, non-professionalised personal support workers (PSWs), who are comparatively poorly paid, minimally trained, often unregulated and less visible, play a key role. In jurisdictions such as Ontario, Canada's largest province, PSWs account for most paid community-based support services such as personal care and homemaking. However, beyond these categories of paid workers exists another, largely uncharted, health human resource universe: untrained, unregulated and mostly invisible unpaid informal carers – the family, friends and neighbours who provide the bulk of everyday care required to support the wellbeing and independence of persons of all ages with ongoing health and social needs in community settings. As Lilly (2011) has commented, if paid health providers constitute the visible tip of the health care iceberg, unpaid informal carers constitute its submerged base. This chapter highlights the growing importance and challenging realities of unpaid informal carers which some observers have also characterised as a 'shadow workforce' (Bookman and Harrington 2007) contributing a vast pool of unpaid labour to individuals who need care.

We highlight two main issues. The first concerns the challenges facing carers themselves. Care needs are rising. While the majority of older persons live well and independently in community settings until the last weeks of life, their numbers are steadily growing, and more are living longer with complex chronic health and social needs requiring ongoing support. In addition, medical advances allow more children and adults with previously life threatening conditions to live outside hospitals, albeit often with extensive continuing care needs. In community settings, unpaid informal carers bear much of the increasing burden of care, including the economic costs of lost paid employment. The second issue concerns the challenges facing policy makers. Even as needs rise, unpaid caregiving is declining. Falling birth rates, smaller families, greater geographic mobility, and the growing participation of women in the paid workforce point towards fewer informal carers providing less care in future. At the same time, carer distress and burnout appear to be climbing, undercutting the willingness of carers to continue to care. These factors suggests a growing 'care gap' that health systems will find difficult and costly to fill (McNeil and Hunter 2014). As a result, policy makers in many countries are now experimenting with a mix of policies and practices aimed at recognising and supporting informal carers.

Policy makers are also grappling with the boundaries between paid 'formal' health care workers such as doctors, nurses and PSWs, and unpaid 'informal carers' (Billings and Leichsenring 2014). Should formal and informal providers have separate, but complementary roles, so that only trained and regulated workers provide 'health care' services such as wound care and injections, while most untrained and unregulated carers provide non-medical support such as toileting and transportation? Alternatively, should formal and informal workers be recognised as increasingly substituting one for the other with a permeable boundary between them? Clearly, this boundary is shifting. As more informal carers perform routine medical procedures, such as suctioning and tracheotomy care, previously within the protected and exclusionary realm of the regulated health professions, health professionals – like primary care doctors in the UK – now write non-medical 'social prescriptions' for gardening and volunteering to address loneliness and to improve mental and physical wellbeing (King's Fund 2018).

We begin by charting the characteristics and contributions of informal carers: who they are, what they do, and how they help to sustain not only individuals requiring ongoing care, but increasingly stretched formal health care systems, including the paid health professionals they employ. We then consider the challenges of caregiving. While caring for others can be personally fulfilling, it can also be physically, emotionally and financially onerous, resulting in carer distress, burnout and withdrawal, as well as a reluctance to take on a caregiving role in the first place. Next, we provide an overview of policies being considered or implemented in different jurisdictions to support informal carers, ranging from cash transfers in the form of caregiver allowances or tax credits to in-kind support services such as respite care, training and counselling, and labour market adjustments like carer work leave. Finally, we ask why, in jurisdictions like Canada, carer support policies have been slow to emerge despite growing recognition by policy makers and researchers of the importance of 'caring for carers'.

A portrait of unpaid, informal carers

Informal carers include family members, friends or networks of multiple informal carers who share ongoing caring responsibilities without pay for a few hours a week or round the clock (Carers UK 2015). Informal carers live inside or outside the household of the person requiring help. They can be neighbours or teenagers looking after parents with a terminal illness, young people caring for siblings with drug addictions, parents looking after children with physical or mental disabilities, or an elderly person caring for a dementia-ridden spouse.

Such unpaid, informal carers make essential contributions to the health and wellbeing of individuals with ongoing health and social care needs. These can include Instrumental Activities of Daily Living (IADLs) related to the need for assistance with mobility in the community, shopping, managing money, maintaining the house, and preparing meals. They may also include more personal Activities of Daily Living (ADLs) such as bathing, toileting, grooming, dressing, and feeding. A growing number of informal carers also provide medical care previously provided by regulated health professionals in hospital settings such as physical therapy, tube feeding and administering medications

(Peckham et al 2014). Although not health care *per se*, the ability to perform IADLs and ADLs is increasingly acknowledged as having a key impact on health and wellbeing, particularly in ageing societies. In its conceptualisation of 'healthy ageing,' defined as maintaining functional capacity 'to do the things we value for as long as possible', the World Health Organization (WHO) (2015a) clarifies that 'disease' is only one of the factors that influences health in older age; non-medical factors such as housing, transportation and social connections play crucial roles. Indeed, in its ground-breaking work on 'age-friendly cities', the WHO highlights the critical importance of non-medical resources such as transportation, housing, social participation and community support in determining health and wellbeing not just for older persons, but for other groups including young women and children who may also face day-to-day challenges (WHO 2007).

Recent data from Canadian cities underscore the importance of non-medical supports to health and wellbeing. To illustrate this, although a majority of older people in Toronto judged their general health as good, very good or excellent, 20 per cent reported difficulties with mobility, including needing equipment to walk, a wheelchair and help from other people. Some 27 per cent also said they needed help with one or more essential daily tasks, including preparing meals, doing housework, personal care, going to appointments, running errands and paying bills (City of Toronto 2017). Moreover, in data from the Organization for Economic Cooperation and Development (OECD) (2017), a group of 34 mostly rich countries indicate that informal carers play a key role in responding to such needs. For example, more than one in ten adults provided help with ADLs, mostly personal care such as grooming, toileting and feeding. If one were also to consider help with the IADLs, one in three adults over 50 provided unpaid care and about 60 per cent of those informal carers were women (Colombo et al 2011; OECD 2017). Most caregiving was for close relatives such as parents or spouses. Moreover, while about half of all carers provided fewer than 10 hours of care per week, most informal carers in countries like Spain and South Korea provided more than 20 hours of care per week.

This international portrait is consistent with data from Canada (Sinha 2013) showing that 46 per cent of Canadians aged 15 and older provided care to a family member or friend with a long-term health condition, disability or ageing needs. Women represented 54 per cent of caregivers and were likely to spend more time per week on caregiving activities than males. Despite their unpaid caring responsibilities, 60 per cent of carers also worked in a paid job or business, with 48 per cent reporting caring for their own parents or parents-in-law over the past year. Other care recipients included friends or neighbours (16 per cent), grandparents (13 per cent), siblings and extended family members (10 per cent), spouses (8 per cent) and sons or daughters (5 per cent). While carers performed a range of tasks, providing transportation was most common at 73 per cent. Additional tasks included housework (51 per cent), house maintenance and outdoor work (45 per cent), scheduling and coordinating appointments (31 per cent), managing finances (27 per cent), and providing personal care (22 per cent). Further, almost a quarter (23 per cent) helped with medical treatments previously provided by health care professionals.

In the UK around one in ten people currently provide unpaid care (Carers Trust 2019). About three in five people will be carers at some point in their lives, and consistent with the international picture, 58 per cent of carers are women. Carers are also workers: one in eight workers (4.27 million people) are carers, while one in five people aged 50 to 60 are carers, with about 65 per cent of carers over 60 years themselves having chronic health problems or a disability. Of all the carers in the UK, 11 per cent look after people with dementia, two-thirds of whom live at home. Almost 1.4 million people provide over 50 hours of unpaid care per week, which does not consider the responsibilities of full-time work, combining caring with looking after young children, or travelling long distances to provide care, all of which can have a serious impact on life (Carers UK 2015). Beyond providing ADLs and IADLs, informal carers also greatly enhance the social quality of life of care recipients. Until recently, policy makers have largely dismissed emotional labour as unimportant and tangential to health compared to practical instrumental tasks. However, social activities such as the cup of tea, spontaneous songs, game of cards or informal conversations accompanying mundane tasks do much to offer vital emotional engagement and companionship. Such interpersonal contact and social connectedness can help relieve a sense of isolation among older people, promoting social and psychological as well as physical wellbeing.

In fact, countries globally are increasingly identifying social isolation and loneliness as a public health concern leading to adverse mental and physical health. A national survey in the United States found that 35 per cent of Americans aged 45 and older experience loneliness. As health declines, the rate of loneliness among midlife and older adults increases: 51 per cent of midlife and older adults who consider their health to be fair or poor are lonely in contrast to 27 per cent who believe their health to be excellent or very good

(Anderson and Thayer 2018). In 2018 the UK government launched its first 'loneliness strategy' with the appointment of the world's first Minister for Loneliness, largely in response to reports that more than 9 million people in the UK experience loneliness to the detriment of their health (Cox Commission on Loneliness 2018; John 2018). Doctors in the UK will be encouraged to write 'social prescriptions' for friendship referring patients to activities that help tackle feelings of emotional isolation (Harris 2018). The rationale is that prescribing patients to take up baking, dancing, creative painting, tai chi or new activity to meet other people will do more than antidepressants to enhance health and wellbeing. The idea of 'social prescriptions' for friendship highlights the critical importance of the spontaneous social interactions that occur during informal caring.

By supporting the health and wellbeing of individuals, carers also help to sustain formal health care systems. A recent Canadian expert report concluded that unpaid caregivers often come to represent the most important members of their care teams and that without their daily contributions, many older adults wishing to age in place would otherwise have to turn to alternative and more institutional residential care settings (Sinha 2012). Another report adds that our health system could not sustain current levels of care in the community without the ongoing contribution of family caregivers (Donner et al 2015); for every two hours of paid care in community settings, unpaid carers contributed an average of seven hours of help. The value of such caregiving contributions is enormous. Canadian carers contribute the equivalent of C$25 billion each year by providing care that hospitals or residential care settings would otherwise have to provide (Carers Canada ND; Hollander et al 2009). Carers contribute an additional C$12.6 million per year in the form of direct out-of-pocket expenses for services such as transportation and homemaking as well as uninsured health care supplies like wheelchairs and other assistive devices, incontinence and other personal hygienic supplies, vitamins and other food supplements, and over-the-counter drugs. As a result, more than 2 million Canadians with ongoing health and social needs can live safely and appropriately outside costly hospitals and residential care. The contributions of carers in other countries are similarly substantial. The Carers Trust (2019) estimates that the economic value of the contribution of carers in the UK is more than the total NHS budget, equivalent to £132 billion every year. As for the United States, the estimated economic value of services provided by informal carers stood at $470 billion in 2013, exceeding the value of paid home care and total Medicaid spending (Reinhard et al 2015).

The challenging realities of caring

As noted earlier, such extensive personal and economic contributions have led some observers to characterise informal carers as the submerged base of the health care iceberg. Other investigators have described carers as a semi-voluntary, conscripted workforce expected to balance unpaid caring with family responsibilities and paid work, with or without formal support (Duxbury et al 2009). Such observations have prompted researchers and policy makers to pay greater attention to the challenging realities faced by unpaid carers and the consequences of a possible decline in caregiving.

Rising and more complex needs

The first challenge concerns the rising needs outside hospitals and other institutional settings – ageing populations, along with medical advances allowing children and adults with previously life threatening conditions to live longer, mean more care is needed closer to home. While much of this relates to demographic shifts as people live longer, deliberate policy changes shortening hospital stays compound the impact. Since the 1990s policy makers in Canada and other industrialised countries have steadily reduced the number of hospital beds, as well as the days patients spend in the remaining beds so people are now discharged 'sicker and quicker' to access care in the community. According to the OECD (2019:1) efficiency and cost containment are major considerations: 'all other things being equal, a shorter stay will reduce the cost per discharge and shift care from inpatient to less expensive post-acute settings'. Of course, home and community settings are less expensive precisely because care is provided mostly by poorly paid workers such as PSWs and by unpaid carers. A shift toward care in the home and out of institutions invariably means even greater reliance on unpaid caregivers.

In addition to a greater volume of care needs, unpaid carers also face increasingly complex needs. Recent data from the Canadian Institute for Health Information (2018) show that more than eight in ten older Canadians rated their own health as 'excellent, very good or good'. However, about a third experienced three or more chronic conditions, including hypertension or high blood pressure, heart disease, diabetes, asthma or chronic lung disease, depression, anxiety or other mental health problems, cancer, joint pain or arthritis, and stroke. This is slightly higher than in countries such as the UK, Sweden and Germany where about 30 per cent of older persons reported multiple chronic conditions, but considerably lower than in the United States where the corresponding number is 44 per cent, the highest in the industrial world. Moreover, around 14 per cent of older Canadians reported depression, anxiety or other mental health problems, as well as chronic medical conditions. About 20 per cent said that they had difficulties coping with emotional distress, and 17 per cent felt isolated from others. Demonstrating how health and social deficits can reinforce one another, older Canadians with lower incomes were considerably more likely than those with higher incomes to report poor health status, distress and needing help.

Rising numbers of older persons with dementia add to the challenges facing unpaid carers. Issues with perception, judgement and memory loss can inhibit the ability of persons with health-related challenges to manage routine tasks and personal care on a daily basis, to interpret their environment, to recognise when they need help, and to access formal health and social care in timely fashion. When neuro-cognitive changes are combined with age-related declines in vision, hearing and mobility, and/or the lack of an informal caregiver, dementia becomes a 'game changer' often requiring 24/7 supervision and support. Dementia is associated with more years of disability than many other chronic illnesses and accounts for a higher burden of illness overall (Morton-Chang et al 2017). System factors too invariably come into play. Fragmented silos of health care increase the stress for carers when they attempt to access and coordinate multiple services for dementia and other chronic conditions from providers across health and social care for care recipients.

Carer costs and consequences

A second challenge concerns the impact of caregiving activities on informal carers. Although informal caregiving has been considered 'free' work, it comes at a cost. While there are many positive aspects related to informal caregiving such as reciprocity of care and personal satisfaction, it can lead to physical, emotional and financial strain as well as caregiver fatigue, ill health and burnout (Duxbury et al 2009). Intensive caregiving, whether for children, frail older persons, adults with physical or mental health challenges or those at the end of life, can result in a range of negative consequences, including limited sleep, reduced participation in social activities, chronic distress, depression, higher rates of back problems, migraine headaches, stomach/intestinal ulcers and chronic pain, withdrawal from paid work, and higher risk of poverty.

To illustrate this, most carers in the UK stated that caring had a negative impact on their physical and mental health, with approximately 28 per cent of carers saying that they had their own physical disabilities (Embracing Carers 2017). Caregiving can limit social engagement while increasing the risks of physical and mental health problems including stress and depression. Carers can also experience work disruptions including loss of income and benefits. Canadian data suggest that, as a result of their caregiving activities, 44 per cent of carers missed days of work; 15 per cent reduced their work hours; and 10 per cent left the labour force as a result of having to quit, being fired or taking early retirement (Carers Canada 2019). Such costs may be on the rise. As caregiving becomes more complex, often crossing into the previously exclusive realm of the regulated health professions, it is also more stressful and demanding. A study in the United States found that 46 per cent of family carers reported they were afraid of making a mistake while performing medical or nursing tasks with little or no training for recipients with multiple chronic physical and cognitive conditions. Tasks included wound care, managing multiple medications, administering intravenous fluids and injections, monitoring blood sugar levels, preparing special diets, and operating medical equipment (Reinhard et al 2012). Growing numbers of persons with dementia can also place additional demands on carers. Compared with caring for non-dementia, those caring for persons with dementia spend more hours providing care and experience greater emotional strain and poorer physical health outcomes (Reinhard et al 2015). The impact on informal caregivers can be severe with many experiencing significant distress as a result (Stall et al 2018).

Unpaid caring in decline

A third challenge relates to waning carer capacity. A key assumption among policy makers in Canada and elsewhere seems to be that that carers will continue to do more for moral and ethical reasons, or simply because there is no alternative (Williams et al 2015). However, this assumption may no longer be true. Demographic and social factors play a major role: birth rates are dropping, families are getting smaller, living arrangements are changing, and women, who still account for the majority of informal caregivers across the industrialised world, are engaged in paid employment outside the home. Moreover, potential carers may be less willing to step up because of the perception that 'free' caregiving work is not valued, and that formal systems will kick in only when caregivers are themselves at the point of crisis.

Although Canada is still a relatively young country compared to Japan, Italy, Greece and Germany, it too is ageing, in part because older Canadians are living longer. Equally important is the fact that birth rates are dropping and there are fewer children to replenish the bottom of the population pyramid. For the first time in 2016, the number of older Canadians (those 65 years and older) exceeded the number of younger Canadians (those 14 years and younger), and the proportion of those aged 15 to 65 years declined (Senate of Canada 2017). These demographics suggest that in future fewer informal carers will be available. Rural and remote areas are often disproportionately affected. Young adults, and potential caregivers, are among the first to leave following education and jobs to cities with older persons staying behind. As a result, New Brunswick, a mostly rural Canadian province, has one of the fastest ageing populations in Canada (Statistics Canada 2015).

Even in urban areas increasing numbers of older persons are living alone. In 2016 just under 30 per cent of Canadians of all ages lived in 'one person' households; by comparison, between 40 per cent and 45 per cent of all older women lived alone (Statistics Canada 2015). In Toronto the numbers were lower but still noteworthy: an estimated 27 per cent of seniors lived alone putting them at risk of poor eating habits, physical inactivity, falls and depression, while also increasing the risk of hospitalisation and death from heart disease, stroke and suicide (City of Toronto 2017). Consider also the impact on emerging communities in urban and other settings. Lesbian, gay, bisexual, transsexual (LGBT) communities may be less likely to have family carers, as they may be distant from their birth families, are less likely to have children, and, in the past, were more likely to have experienced the death of a partner to HIV/AIDS (Brotman and Ryan 2009; Grossman et al 2000). Many industrialised countries are experiencing similar trends with profound implications at individual and system levels. In the UK McNeil and Hunter (2014) concluded that, even as care needs grow, in part because of an ageing population, the supply of carers is likely to produce a growing 'care gap' as the number of older persons needing care outstrips the number of family members able to provide it, in turn placing a greater burden on fewer carers.

The policy response: caring for caregivers

Even as the contributions and challenges faced by informal caregivers become more apparent, policy makers remain divided in their responses. Choice of support varies widely, from formal recognition to in-kind services such as respite and homemaking, to cash transfers such as carers' allowances and tax credits, and workplace policies that allow carers to take paid or unpaid work leave. In addition, some jurisdictions like the UK, Germany and Japan are now implementing wide-ranging innovations aimed at building new social institutions such as intergenerational housing that redefine caring relationships, while blurring the strict boundary between paid health care workers and unpaid carers.

Carer recognition

A first step taken by some jurisdictions is to recognise informal carers officially. Although recognition in itself may not directly reduce the care burden, it acknowledges carers as active participants, if not full partners, in care delivery alongside, and often in collaboration with, paid health care providers. In Canada, carers are only slowly gaining public recognition. Manitoba was the first to enact a Caregiver Recognition Act in 2011. It acknowledges informal carers in their own right, establishes an annual Caregiver Recognition Day, provides a framework for a Caregiver Advisory Committee to the Minister of Healthy Living and Seniors, and sets out general principles for government and agencies to consult with, and support, caregivers (Legislative Assembly of Manitoba 2011). Ontario is promoting 'engagement' between health professionals and informal carers. Health Quality Ontario (2019), a quasi-government organisation tasked with developing evidence-based standards for care, has published data demonstrating the extent of carer contributions to persons with ongoing home care needs, and the distress that many carers experience as a result. It encourages caregiver training, education and participation in home and community care and across the health care system. Quebec has also formalised caregiving recognition. In 2018 it created a Minister Responsible for Seniors and Informal Caregivers. This Minister will be the first Cabinet-level appointment in Canada that recognises carers in their own right (National Assembly of Quebec 2018).

Carer support and advocacy networks

In many countries carer support networks are emerging, often subsidised in part by government, to connect carers to counselling, education and support services, to advocate the expansion of carer support policies, and to redefine relationships between unpaid carers and paid care workers. For example, Carers Canada (2019) is a national coalition of diverse national and local organisations connecting carers with providers as well as policy makers and other stakeholders to advocate progressive carer support policies. Carers UK (2014a) is a national network that connects carers to a range of supports and promotes carer support policies. In consultation with carers, the network developed an innovative 'app' called 'Jointly' that allows the circle of professional and unpaid carers of care recipients to share information in a single messaging system. 'Jointly' becomes the place to record health logs, track medications, and monitor who is doing what on which days. The app facilitates access to system navigators who can help carers find the appropriate providers as smoothly as possible, as well as professionals who can provide education, training, and information (Carers UK 2014b).

In the United States several carer support networks have emerged. The Caregiver Action Network (2017) provides practical help, support and information to a broad spectrum of family carers ranging from the parents of children with special needs, to the families and friends of wounded soldiers, to adult children caring for parents with Alzheimer's disease. Similarly, ARCH National Respite Network and Resource Center (2017) is a non-profit organisation which provides a searchable, online, state-by-state guide to respite service providers and sources of funding to help pay for care. The National Alliance for Caregiving (2019) is a coalition of organisations focusing on advancing family caregiving through research, innovation, and advocacy. Its mission is to recognise the important social and financial contributions of family carers, and to improve quality of life for carers and their families. The Alliance works with other caregiving associations to conduct research, develop national best practice programmes, work to increase public awareness of family caregiving issues, and advance policies that help carers address their challenges.

In Europe, France has Local Centres of Information and Co-ordination in which social workers can provide information and help to individuals on a regular basis on topics related to the needs of older people. These centres also link carers with medical staff to address questions related to the disability of the care recipient (Colombo et al 2011). A broader European organisation, Eurocarers (2019), is an activist network bringing together carer organisations as well as universities and research institutes to advance evidence-based advocacy. It aims to ensure that European Union and national policies take into account the support and services carers need to enable them to remain active in paid employment and to maintain a social life. Meanwhile Carers Australia (2019) is a national body that works directly with state and territory carer associations to improve the wellbeing of its 2.7 million carers, forming 12 per cent of the population, through peer support, counselling, and advice, including 'resources for culturally and linguistically diverse communities' that have been translated into six different languages.

Financial support

A number of countries – including the UK, New Zealand, Sweden, Finland, France, Germany and Australia – have been at the forefront in providing a means-tested 'Carer's Allowance' (Colombo et al 2011; Government of the United Kingdom 2019). Cash allowances paid directly to carers can help them avoid financial distress due to the direct costs of caring or loss of income resulting from having to reduce or leave paid employment. Canada also recently consolidated and simplified its income tax credit system for carers. In its 2017 budget the federal government introduced a 'Canada Caregiver Credit' to provide financial help for caregivers (Government of Canada 2019). The policy provides a tax credit against a carer's income, which increases the allowable income, but only for those caregivers who pay income tax. However, the poorest caregivers, or those who have given up work completely to provide care, receive little financial relief. Importantly, the programme excludes payment to people who provide care to friends. At a provincial level, the Government of Nova Scotia (2015) was an early adopter of direct cash payments to carers. It offers cash payments of C\$400 per month to low-income carers of persons with high levels of impairment or disabilities to help cover financial costs. The province has recently expanded the programme to include carers of individuals with such issues as moderate memory loss, challenging behaviours and a high risk of falls (Laroche 2018).

Work leave

In addition to their unpaid caregiving, many carers work outside the family home, sometimes resulting in unmanageable workloads. In the UK, for example, 4.27 million carers are of working age, where one in five carers have given up employment to provide care. The employment rate for carers is 67 per cent: 72 per cent for men and 62 per cent for women (Carers Trust 2019). Belgium, France, Spain, Ireland, The Netherlands, Austria and Germany have introduced paid and unpaid work leave – time off work for caregiving with a guarantee that carers will not lose their jobs. Yet, even where such policies are in place, benefits tend to be restricted. For example, time off for caring may be relatively short (a few weeks in duration) or limited to carers of children or family members (Colombo et al 2011). Belgium provides the longest paid leave, for a maximum of 12 months, which employers may refuse only on serious business grounds. In Japan paid leave is also comparatively long – up to 93 days with 40 per cent of wages paid through employment insurance if the company does not compensate during the leave. Scandinavian countries tend to pay most in remuneration. For instance, in Norway and Sweden paid leave is equivalent to 100 per cent and 80 per cent of the worker's wage respectively. In Denmark, in exchange for employers continuing to pay full wages during care leave, municipalities reimburse a minimum equivalent to 82 per cent of the sick benefit ceiling.

By contrast, the United States does not guarantee paid leave for family caregiving responsibilities federally and employment protections for family carers are weak and uneven across states. In addition, federal law does not explicitly prohibit discrimination based on caregiver status. As a result, employers may dismiss workers who take time off to care for ill family members; demand that employees drop an ill family member from coverage in the employer's insurance plan; or deny leave for caregiving (Williams et al 2012).

Respite

Carer respite, or time off from caregiving, can alleviate the burden and allow carers to attend to other areas of their lives, including their own health and wellbeing. Respite may be particularly important where care recipients have dementia or other complex care needs requiring 24/7 attention. Respite can take many forms. For instance, home support workers can come to the client's own home to provide relief for the carer. Alternatively, clients can stay in a residential or nursing home and receive dedicated care and attention. Day programmes, operated largely by non-profit organisations, offer activities for care recipients for several hours during the day, from one to five days a week, for a small fee to cover the cost of a meal and transportation.

Access to respite varies widely among OECD countries (Colombo et al 2011). In Canada, while respite is a component of all publicly funded home care programmes, it is not a designated core service and access is not guaranteed. In some jurisdictions, users pay no direct cost for respite at home, while other jurisdictions assess income or income plus assets to determine the proportion of costs, which the family must pay. All jurisdictions except Nunavut require the client to pay a portion of the cost of respite in facilities, with the amount depending on income. A high proportion of those requiring respite are the elderly spouses of elderly clients. Respite in the UK falls under the now updated Care Act 2014, which made provisions to support adults and their carers while devolving the administrative responsibility to local authorities. Social services or social work departments in local councils in England, Wales and Scotland and the local Health and Social Care Trust in Northern Ireland help carers arrange for respite care. To qualify for respite, carers undergo an assessment that considers the impact of caring on their health, wellbeing, work, study, relationships, social activities, goals and housing. Following this assessment, care recipients are also financially assessed to determine whether (and if so, how much) they need to contribute towards respite. The social services/social work department may choose to give direct cash payments to care recipients to arrange and pay for their own care and support while the carer takes a break (Carers UK 2018; Government of the United Kingdom 2019). The 2006 Lifespan Respite Care Act in the United States was designed to address respite issues for families caring for children and adults with special needs (Rose et al 2015). The law awards competitive grants of up to $200,000 to eligible state agencies to create lifespan respite programmes at the state and local levels. The agencies receive funding to offer planned and emergency respite for family caregivers, training/recruitment of respite workers and volunteers, provision of information to caregivers about respite/ support services, assistance for caregivers in gaining access to such services, and the establishment of a National Resource Center on Lifespan Respite Care (Napili and Colello 2013).

Human rights protection

To advance the development of carer support policies, some advocates in Canada have called for establishing carer rights as a basic human right. This call gained momentum in Canada when the Canadian Human Rights Commission (2014) released its document entitled *A Guide to Balancing Work and Caregiving Obligations: Collaborative Approaches for a Supportive and Well-performing Workplace*. Under human rights legislation, employers must accommodate employees who are also carers. Employees on their part must demonstrate that they are obligated to provide care and that it is not simply a matter of personal choice. If they have exhausted reasonable options and alternatives to arrange for the care of their family members, employers are obligated to accommodate the employees on the grounds of 'family status' and consider each employee's request and specific circumstances individually to the point of 'undue hardship'. While there is no precise legal definition of undue hardship or standard formula for determining it, employers must provide concrete evidence as to how the accommodation amounts to 'undue hardship'. However, the grounds for protection remain narrow. Family status still only refers to the parent–child relationship, thereby excluding caring for other family members such as a brother or sister or close friends as in the case of members of the LGBT community who rely on friends and their 'family of choice' for their care. In this regard, advocacy organisations are calling on the Federal and Provincial Governments in Canada to amend their human rights legislation to include 'care' as a protected ground of discrimination in the area of employment to ensure that all carers have human rights protection (Chun and Gallagher-Louisy 2018).

Building and adapting social structures

Some countries such as the UK, Germany and Japan are now looking beyond the individual and family structures. They aim to strengthen collective capacity by building 'new community institutions' and adapting 'social structures already in place' (McNeil and Hunter 2014). An often-cited example is the City of Leeds in the UK (WHO 2015b). Since 2005 each local area in Leeds has had a Neighbourhood Network that helps older people and families get assistance with everyday needs such as free or cheap transport, social activities, shopping, help at home, cleaning, gardening and breaks for carers. These networks also act as gateways for advice, information and services to help older persons live independently, while promoting active civic engagement – one of the WHO's criteria for 'active ageing'. Local management committees including older persons and members of the local community run the networks, including non–health care partners such as charities, community groups, faith-based institutions and volunteers.

Another movement gaining traction is co-housing. Based on the idea of mutual support, growing numbers of models in the UK, Europe, Canada and Australia offer shared living spaces for people who wish to enjoy the benefits of a close-knit community, where all residents contribute, while maintaining the possibility of privacy in their own houses or apartments. Common spaces for activities such as gardening, dancing, lectures, watching movies or physical exercise foster a supportive milieu, where neighbours can help one another (Pedersen 2015). A novel variant is intergenerational co-housing matching younger people seeking affordable housing with older people who wish to stay in their own homes, but need help with chores (CBC News 2018).

Many innovations emphasising broad-scale mutual support have emerged too from 'super ageing' Japan covered more extensively in Chapter eleven. Here those aged 65 or over account for more than 30 per cent of its total population including almost 5 million with dementia. Such advances gained impetus from the national government's plan to have an integrated community-based long-term care system by 2025. The 2015 'New Orange Plan' for dementia care recognises the need to remove institutional barriers between professional providers and informal carers, while backing intergenerational projects of mutual support (Japan Health Policy NOW 2018). Good examples are the 'Dementia Supporters' or 'Dementia Friends' who include over 6 million volunteers mobilised and trained to support people with fading cognitive abilities. 'Dementia Supporters' include well older people who become peer supporters for their frailer counterparts; school children who have been taught what to do when they see seniors appearing lost; store clerks who help when they notice customers walking back and forth in the aisles; garbage collectors who realise an older resident is no longer putting out recycling material; bank tellers who have clients returning to withdraw money for a third time in one day; and apartment managers who deal with elderly tenants knocking on the wrong doors, failing to sort bins, or taking other residents' newspapers (Hayashi 2017).

Recently, in the commercial sector in Japan, some stores have re-imagined their business plans to meet the growing demands of elderly people and their carers (Japan Times 2018). For those who want healthy food and prefer to eat at home, these stores deliver cooking ingredients or small sized, pre-packaged nutritious meals. The drivers deliver food and friendship: they live in the neighbourhood, know their customers, and can have a friendly chat while monitoring the older person's wellbeing. Family Mart is experimenting with sharing space with drug stores so that older people and their carers can do most of their shopping in one location. If tired, a person can rest in a comfortable social meeting space designed for gathering, chatting, eating, and drinking – good for business and convenient for older customers. In 2018 Lawson opened drop-in health care spaces in shops in Tokyo and Kobe so that customers could consult with health experts about their diet and nursing care, and receive needs assessments and support from municipal workers. They also provide free cancer screening in mobile medical centres, free health check-ups without an appointment, facilities to pay public utilities bills, send mail or withdraw money through ATM services (Fujibuchi 2018). Seven-Eleven, Lawson, and FamilyMart have also signed an agreement with Japan's Urban Renaissance Agency to open stores in the agency's apartment complexes. In addition to the same elderly-friendly features as in other branches, the stores will add services such as room cleaning and mending – and may also handle maintenance problems at nights and weekends (Kirk 2016).

Conclusion

Health care systems in the 21st century are undergoing a major transformation as more care shifts from hospitals to home and community. Although comparatively well paid, highly trained, highly regulated and highly visible professionals such as doctors, nurses, technologists and therapists continue to play the lead role in hospitals, the providers fundamentally change outside their walls. As this book reminds us, it is the comparatively poorly paid, trained and regulated PSWs who provide the bulk of paid care in the community, a reality highlighted by worsening worker shortages across Canada and in other countries. Even beyond these paid workers, however, are the unpaid, untrained and mostly invisible informal carers. While policy makers and researchers tend to be preoccupied with the visible tip of the health care iceberg, populated by hospitals and health care professionals, a growing body of international evidence shows that, in addition to paid PSWs, unpaid informal carers constitute the iceberg's base. They are the ones providing most of the ongoing support required to maintain the physical and social health, wellbeing and independence of growing numbers of persons of all ages with ongoing care needs. Moreover, this mostly uncharted base keeps formal health care systems afloat particularly as illnesses that could once be cured on a short-term episodic basis in hospitals are superseded by complex combinations of chronic health and social needs, which must be managed over the long term where people live.

Yet, there are growing concerns that this base may be eroding. Historically, most unpaid carers were family members. But now birth rates are plunging, new social arrangements including living alone are replacing families, and women are increasingly choosing careers over traditional roles in the family home. Moreover, current carers are experiencing substantial costs resulting from their caring activities; in addition to being more prone to physical and mental health disorders, carers may also experience a significant economic burden due to lost income and out-of-pocket expenses. Such costs contribute to rising levels of distress, burnout and withdrawal for current carers, while discouraging future carers to step up. For policy makers now waking up to the pivotal role played by unpaid carers in supporting people and sustaining formal care systems, there seems to be a growing consensus that something needs to be done.

There is, however, less consensus on exactly what to do. Various OECD countries have implemented different combinations of carer support policies and programmes, but without systematic evaluation of costs or outcomes, many questions remain unanswered (Williams et al 2015). Which supports are most likely to encourage current carers to continue and future caregivers to step in? Could carer supports also persuade carers to do less, since they may think that government will do it for them? In countries such as Canada, carer support policies have been slow to emerge. In part, this policy reluctance reflects the focus on hospital-centred curative medical care (OECD 2017). It also reflects the tough political reality that, particularly in periods of constrained budgets, resources for carers will almost certainly have to be diverted from hospitals and health professionals. Moreover, in recognising the vital but often invisible role of unpaid carers, as well as paid PSWs, policy makers also have to consider the consequences of a further blurring of the lines between highly trained and regulated health care professionals like doctors and nurses and less well trained and regulated formal and informal carers. As we have seen, a substantial proportion of informal carers now perform routine medical procedures previously within the protected and exclusionary realm of health professions. On the other hand, more health professionals, such as general practitioners in the UK, now see the value of non-medical 'social prescriptions' to address loneliness and improve mental and physical wellbeing in the community.

Finally, the many exciting innovations in Japan, Germany and elsewhere redraw the lines between carers and care recipients by recasting the challenges of ageing and other populations as a collective, rather than as an individual, problem. By emphasising the principles of mutual support and assistance among people, across generations and communities, such innovations diminish the 'top-down' hierarchical relationships that characterise formal health care systems and acknowledge that carers may also be care recipients and vice versa. Just as importantly, these innovations shift the policy focus from the delivery of conventional, provider-driven health care services, to the needs of individuals and communities. Here, the evidence is unequivocal: while health care systems are good at curing illnesses, they are poorly equipped to promote health and social wellbeing – for which the hitherto relatively invisible role of unpaid informal carers is critical, alongside paid health support workers, in the health care division of labour (Saks and Allsop 2007).

References

Anderson, G.O. and Thayer, C.E. (2018) *A National Survey of Adults 45 and Older: Loneliness and Social Connections*, Washington, DC: AARP, www.aarp.org/content/dam/aarp/research/surveys_statistics/life-leisure/2018/loneliness-social-connections-2018.doi.10.26419-2Fres.00246.001.pdf

ARCH National Respite Network and Resource Center (2017) *ABCs of Respite: A Consumer's Guide for Family Caregivers*, Chapel Hill, NC, https://archrespite.org/images/docs/ABCs_of_Respite/ABCsofRespite_Updated_6-17.pdf

Billings, J. and Leichsenring, K. (2014) 'Methodological development of the interactive INTERLINKS Framework for Long-term Care,' *International Journal of Integrated Care* 14(2): 1–10.

Bookman, A. and Harrington, M. (2007) 'Family caregivers: A shadow workforce in the geriatric healthcare system', *Journal of Health Politics, Policy and Law* 32(6): 1005–41.

Brotman, S. and Ryan, B. (2009) *Healthy Aging for Gay and Lesbian Seniors in Canada: An Environmental Scan*, Montreal: McGill University, School of Social Work, www.rainbowhealthontario.ca/resources/healthy-aging-for-gay-and-lesbian-seniors-in-canada/

Canadian Human Rights Commission (2014) *A Guide To Balancing Work and Caregiving Obligations: Collaborative Approaches for a Supportive and Well-performing Workplace*, Ottawa: Minister of Public Works and Government Services, www.chrc-ccdp.gc.ca/eng/content/guide-balancing-work-and-caregiving-obligations

Canadian Institute for Health Information. (2018) *How Canada Compares: Results from the Commonwealth Fund's 2017 International Health Policy Survey of Seniors*, Ottawa: CIHI, www.cihi.ca/sites/default/files/document/commonwealth-survey-2017-chartbook-en-rev2-web.pptx

Caregiver Action Network (2017) 'Take Care', https://caregiveraction.org/take-care-august-2017

Carers Australia. (2019) 'About Us', www.carersaustralia.com.au/about-us/

Carers Canada (2019) 'A Canadian Caregiver Strategy', www.carerscanada.ca/priorities/#caregiver-strategy

Carers Canada (ND) 'Carer Facts', www.carerscanada.ca/carer-facts/

Carers Trust (2019) 'Key Facts about Carers and the People They Care for', https://carers.org/key-facts-about-carers-and-people-they-care

Carers UK (2014a) 'About Us', www.carersuk.org/about-us

Carers UK (2014b) 'Jointly App', www.carersuk.org/search/jointly-app

Carers UK (2015) 'Facts about carers', *Policy Briefing*, October, www.carersuk.org/images/Facts_about_Carers_2015.pdf

Carers UK (2018) *Taking a Break*, London: Carers UK, www.carersuk.org/images/Carers_UK_Taking_a_break_UK-wide_UK1016_1118_web_version.pdf

CBC News (2018) 'My Home Was Their Home: Why Seniors, Students Living Together Saves More than Rent Money', 22 July, www.cbc.ca/news/canada/toronto/intergenerational-home-sharing-pilot-program-1.4757060

Chamberlain, J.M., Dent, M. and Saks, M. (eds) (2018) *Professional Health Regulation in the Public Interest: International Perspectives*, Bristol: Policy Press.

Chun, J., and Gallagher-Louisy, C. (2018) *Overview of Human Rights Codes by Province and Territory in Canada*, Ottawa: Canadian Centre for Diversity and Inclusion, https://ccdi.ca/media/1414/20171102-publications-overview-of-hr-codes-by-province-final-en.pdf

City of Toronto (2017) *Healthy Aging in Toronto*, www.toronto.ca/legdocs/mmis/2017/hl/bgrd/backgroundfile-101655.pdf

Collins, S.M., Wacker, R.R. and Roberto, K.A. (2013) 'Considering quality of life for older adults: A view from two countries', *Generations* 37(1): 80–6.

Colombo, F., Llena-Nozal, A., Mercier, J. and Tjadens, F. (2011) *Help Wanted? Providing and Paying for Long-Term Care*, OECD Health Policy Studies, Paris: OECD Publishing, www.oecd-ilibrary.org/social-issues-migration-health/help-wanted_9789264097759-en

Cox Commission on Loneliness (2018) *Combating Loneliness One Conversation at a Time: A Call to Action*, London, www.jocoxloneliness.org/

Donner, G., McReynolds, J., Smith, K., Fooks, C., Sinha, S. and Thomson, D. (2015) *Bringing Care Home. Report of the Expert Group on Home and Community Care*, Report of the Expert Group on Home and Community Care, http://health.gov.on.ca/en/public/programs/lhin/docs/hcc_report.pdf

Duxbury, L., Higgins, C. and Schroeder, B. (2009) *Balancing Paid Work and Caregiving Responsibilities: A Closer Look at Family Caregivers in Canada*, http://observgo.uquebec.ca/observgo/fichiers/37864_PSOC-9.pdf

Embracing Carers (2017) *2017 Carers Report: Embracing the Critical Role of Caregivers around the World – White Paper and Action Plan*, Darmstadt: Merck KGaA, www.embracingcarers.com/content/dam/web/healthcare/corporate/embracing-carers/media/infographics/us/Merck%20KGaA%20Embracing%20Carers_White%20Paper%20Flattened.pdf

Eurocarers (2019) 'About Us', www.eurocarers.org/

Fujibuchi, S. (2018) 'Lawson store in Tokyo opens health care corner staffed by experts', *Mainichi*, 2 August, https://mainichi.jp/english/articles/20180802/p2a/00m/0na/019000c

Government of Canada (2019) 'The Canada Caregiver Credit', www.canada.ca/en/revenue-agency/services/tax/individuals/topics/about-your-tax-return/tax-return/completing-a-tax-return/deductions-credits-expenses/canada-caregiver-amount.html

Government of Nova Scotia (2015) *Living Well: Continuing Care Services*, https://novascotia.ca/dhw/ccs/documents/Living-Wel-%20Continuing-Care-Services.pdf

Government of the United Kingdom (2019) 'Carer's Allowance', www.gov.uk/carers-allowance

Grossman, A.H., D'Augelli, A.R. and Hershberger, S.L. (2000) 'Social support networks of lesbian, gay, and bisexual adults 60 years of age and older', *Journals of Gerontology Series B* 55(3): 171–9.

Harris, B. (2018) 'Doctors in the UK are prescribing social activities to fight against loneliness', World Economic Forum, 19 February, www.weforum.org/agenda/2018/02/line-dancing-and-baking-a-prescription-for-good-health/

Hayashi, M. (2017) 'The Dementia Friends Initiative – Supporting people with dementia and their carers: Reflections from Japan', *International Journal of Care and Caring* 1(2): 281–87.

Health Quality Ontario (2019) 'Patient and family advisors: Coming together to transform the health system', www.hqontario.ca/Events/Health-Quality-Transformation-2015/Patient-and-Family-Advisors-Coming-Together-to-Transform-the-Health-System

Hollander, M.J., Guiping, L. and Chappell, N.L. (2009) 'Who cares and how much? The imputed economic contribution to the Canadian healthcare system of middle-aged and older unpaid caregivers providing care to the elderly', *Healthcare Quarterly* 12(2): 42–9.

Japan Health Policy NOW (2018) *Dementia*, http://japanhpn.org/wp-content/uploads/2018/11/JHPN_Dementia_ENG_20181122_vFinal.pdf

Japan Times (2018) 'Convenience stores tap into health boom', 27 January, www.japantimes.co.jp/life/2018/01/27/food/convenience-stores-tap-health-boom/#.XK5GUmW1a8F.email

John, T. (2018) 'How the world's first loneliness minister will tackle the sad reality of modern life', *Time London*, 25 April, http://time.com/5248016/tracey-crouch-uk-loneliness-minister/

King's Fund (2018) 'Social prescribing: Coming of age', www.kingsfund.org.uk/events/social-prescribing

Kirk, M. (2016) 'How 7-elevens are becoming lifelines for Japan's elderly', *CityLab*, 1 August, www.citylab.com/life/2016/08/how-7-elevens-are-becoming-lifelines-for-japans-elderly/493772/

Laroche, J. (2018) 'More people eligible for caregiver allowance, but no change to amount', *CBC News*, www.cbc.ca/news/canada/nova-scotia/caregiver-allowance-nova-scotia-ns-health-impairment-1.4574295

Legislative Assembly of Manitoba (2011) *Bill 42: The Caregiver Recognition Act, 2011*, https://web2.gov.mb.ca/bills/39-5/pdf/b042.pdf

Lilly, M. (2011) *Who Really Cares? Caregiving Intensity, Labour Supply and Policymaking in Canada*, www.queensu.ca/sps/sites/webpublish.queensu.ca.spswww/files/files/Events/Conferences/QIISP/2011/meredith_lilly.pdf

McNeil, C. and Hunter J. (2014) *The Generation Strain: Collective Solutions to Care in an Ageing Society*, Institute for Public Policy Research, www.ippr.org/publications/the-generation-strain-collective-solutions-to-care-in-an-ageing-society

Morton-Chang, F., Williams, A.P., Berta, W. and Laporte, A. (2017) 'Toward a community-based dementia care strategy: How do we get there from here?', *HealthcarePapers* 16(2): 8–32.

Napili, A. and Colello, K.J. (2013) *Funding for the Older Americans Act and Other Aging Services Programs*, Washington, DC: Congressional Research Service, https://fas.org/sgp/crs/misc/RL33880.pdf

National Alliance for Caregiving (2019) 'About the Alliance', www.caregiving.org/about/about-the-alliance/

National Assembly of Quebec (2018) 'Marguerite Blais, Minister Responsible for Seniors and Informal Caregivers', www.assnat.qc.ca/en/deputes/blais-marguerite-1263/index.html

OECD (2017) *Health at a Glance 2017: OECD Indicators*, Paris: OECD Publishing, http://dx.doi.org/10.1787/health_glance-2017-en

OECD (2019) *Length of Hospital Stay (Indicator): OECD Data*, Paris: OECD Publishing, https://data.oecd.org/healthcare/length-of-hospital-stay.html

Peckham, A., Spalding, K., Watkins, J., Bruce-Barrett, C., Grasic, M. and Williams, A.P. (2014) 'Caring for caregivers of high needs children', *Health Care Quarterly* 17(3): 30–5.

Pedersen, M. (2015) 'Senior co-housing communities in Denmark', *Journal of Housing for the Elderly* 29(1–2): 126–45.

Reinhard, S.C., Levine, C. and Samis, S. (2012) 'Home alone: Family caregivers providing complex Chronic Care', *AARP Public Policy Institute,* Washington, DC: AARP, www.aarp.org/content/dam/aarp/research/public_policy_institute/health/home-alone-family-caregivers-providing-complex-chronic-care-rev-AARP-ppi-health.pdf

Reinhard, S.C., Feinberg, L.F., Choula, R. and Houser, A. (2015) 'Valuing the invaluable: 2015 update', *AARP Public Policy Institute,* Washington DC: AARP, www.aarp.org/content/dam/aarp/ppi/2015/valuing-the-invaluable-2015-update-new.pdf

Rose, M.S., Noelker, L.S. and Kagan, J. (2015) 'Improving policies for caregiver respite services', *The Gerontologist* 55(2): 302–308.

Saks, M. (2010) 'Analyzing the professions: The case for the neo-Weberian approach', *Comparative Sociology* 9(6): 887–915.

Saks, M. and Allsop, J. (2007) 'Social policy, professional regulation and health support work in the United Kingdom', *Social Policy and Society* 6(2): 165–77.

Schulz, R. and Martire, L.M. (2004) 'Family caregiving of persons with dementia: Prevalence, health effects, and support strategies', *American Journal of Geriatric Psychiatry* 12(3): 240–9.

Senate of Canada (2017) *Getting Ready: For a New Generation of Active Seniors,* Report of the Standing Senate Committee on National Finance, Ottawa, https://sencanada.ca/content/sen/committee/421/NFFN/Reports/NFFN_Final19th_Aging_e.pdf

Sinha, M. (2013) *Portrait of Caregivers, 2012,* Ottawa, Canada: Statistics Canada, Catalogue no. 89-652-X, www150.statcan.gc.ca/n1/pub/89-652-x/89-652-x2013001-eng.pdf

Sinha, S. (2012) *Living Longer, Living Well: Recommendations to Inform a Seniors Strategy for Ontario,* www.health.gov.on.ca/en/common/ministry/publications/reports/seniors_strategy/docs/seniors_strategy_report.pdf

Stall, N.M., Sanghum, J.K., Hardacre, K.A., Shah, P.S., Straus, S.E., Bronskill, S.E., Lix, L., Bell, C.M. and Rochon, P.A. (2018) 'Association of informal caregiver distress with health outcomes of community-dwelling care recipients: A systematic review', *Journal of American Geriatric Society* 67(3): 609–17.

Starr, P. (1982) *The Social Transformation of American Medicine: The Rise of a Sovereign Profession and the Making of a Vast Industry*, New York: Basic Books.

Statistics Canada (2015) 'Percentage of the population aged 15 and over living alone by age group, Canada, 2001 and 2011', *Living Arrangements of Seniors: Families, Households and Marital Status, Structural Type of Dwelling and Collectives, 2011 Census of Population*, www12. statcan.gc.ca/census-recensement/2011/as-sa/98-312-x/98-312-x2011003_4-eng.pdf

Williams, A.P., Peckham, A., Kuluski K., Lum, J., Warrick, N., Spalding, K., Tam, T., Bruce-Barrett, C., Grasic, M. and Im, J. (2015) 'Caring for caregivers: Challenging the assumptions', *Healthcare Papers* 15(1): 8–21.

Williams, J.C., Devaux, R., Petrac, P. and Feinberg, L. (2012) 'Protecting family caregivers from employment discrimination,' *AARP Public Policy Institute, INSIGHT on the Issues 68*, Washington, DC, www.aarp.org/content/dam/aarp/research/public_policy_institute/health/protecting-caregivers-employment-discrimination-insight-AARP-ppi-ltc.pdf

World Health Organization (2007) *Global Age-friendly Cities: A Guide*, www.who.int/ageing/publications/Global_age_friendly_cities_Guide_English.pdf

World Health Organization (2015a) *Aging and Health*, www.who.int/ageing/events/world-report-2015-launch/healthy-ageing-infographic.jpg?ua=1

World Health Organization (2015b) *Making Leeds the Best City to Grow Old*, https://extranet.who.int/agefriendlyworld/making-leeds-the-best-city-to-grow-old-2/

FOUR

The management and leadership of support workers

Mike Dent

Introduction

Support workers in health and social care increasingly cover a wide range of activities which can include patients and clients' self-management, through voluntary and family care support networks (Jeffries et al 2015; Milligan 2018). This is in addition to paid support workers within the private as well as public sectors, the former playing a particularly large role in the provision of care homes for the elderly. While support work covers a whole range of activities in these sectors and associated domains, including in private family settings, attention in this chapter will be restricted to institutionalised contexts within health and social care including hospitals, clinics, care homes and residential homes. It is here that problems of management and leadership have been most strongly identified and attempts made to address them. In terms of terminology, as in the rest of the volume, 'support work' and 'support workers' will be used as a generic term covering both the health and social care sectors, while explicit differentiation will be made between the specific categories of support work in health care and social care where necessary in the text.

This chapter will focus on the following key developments, particularly as they relate to the issues of the management and leadership of support workers based on a neo-Weberian approach to professions and professionalisation:

- The New Public Management (NPM) and the professional upgrading/reorientation of nursing and the reinvention of support workers.
- The initial implications and further consequences of this trend for support workers and their management.

- The shift from the NPM towards the New Public Governance (NPG) and a leadership approach as a means of resolving the challenges of controlling and coordinating support workers.
- The question of the putative professionalisation of support workers, given the changing dynamics of professionalism and professionalisation in the public and private sector.

The chapter will predominantly focus on developments related to nursing in the UK as an exemplar. It will also draw on evidence from across the European continent to elaborate on various points and to ensure the account is not too myopically Anglo-centric.

The New Public Management and professionalism in health and social care

The key to understanding the dynamics of the health and social care professions and the processes of professionalisation today lies largely in being aware of the impact that the NPM has had on these occupations and others that overlap with them in the division of labour. Specifically, the NPM is crucially relevant to the expansion of the support work labour force in the health and social care sectors and its organisation and management. The process has been driven by a neo-liberal agenda with the intention to contain the costs of public sector health and social care (Dent 2015). It can be said to have two aspects. First, it is a doctrine on how private business concepts, techniques and values would make the public sector, including health and social care, more efficient (Pollitt and Bouckaert 2011). In the present context, this was to be achieved principally by the privatisation of social and health care facilities and/or contracting out of services (Kirkpatrick 2006; Pollock 2005). Second, it is a direct approach to the control and coordination of the work organisation, be it a care home, hospital or clinic. Hood (1991, 1995) notably summarised this aspect early on in the implementation of the NPM. It was seen as replacing public sector administration with a business style of management within a competitive environment (whether privatised or not) and being aided by providing user choice of service provider. Internally there was to be more direct *management* intervention in what had been *professionally* dominated organisations, and with it a strong downward pressure on costs and resource use. This was to be further supported by a heavy emphasis on performance targets and outcome measures (Klein 2013).

The NPM radically changed the administration of the public services across Europe from the 1980s onwards (Christensen and

Laegreid 2011; Pollitt and Bouckaert 2011). It was adopted in the UK earlier than in other European countries, although Scandinavia – in particular, Sweden – was also an early adopter. The neo-liberal policy thinking initially driving the NPM is reflected in it taking root within those countries most influenced by this – especially Thatcherite Britain. However, it also appealed to other tax-funded health and social care systems experiencing political pressures to contain costs within these sectors, as in the case of Sweden (Dent 2003b). The Southern European countries – for example, Italy and Greece – also embraced the NPM fairly early on, although their particular 'path dependencies' (Dent et al 2012; Wilsford 1994) tended to mean the trajectory taken by NPM policies in health and social care in impacting on the role of support work was notably dissimilar to the pattern in Northern Europe. These Southern European variants have been far more influenced by the local dynamics of 'familialism' (Dent 2005), which has meant that the health and social care sectors have been underdeveloped in comparison to their counterparts in Northern Europe and Scandinavia. This is in part because it has been the common expectation within Southern European countries that the family will take on far more of the responsibility for health and social care than in other Western countries (Dent 2003a; Marí-Klose and Moreno-Fuentes 2013; Trifiletti 1999).

Health and social care in continental European countries is based more on a hypothecated funding system historically based on sickness funds – a statutory health insurance, which also covered social care to a greater or lesser extent (Robinson, Gregory and Jabbal 2014). Over recent decades this health insurance-based system has been largely marketised (that is, privatised) in the belief that the competition this would introduce would result in greater efficiencies within the systems. This reflects the logic of the NPM as applied to the 'sickness fund' model (Dent 2003b). Although there is a *prima facie* similarity to the United States (also a health insurance-based system), in Europe there is a much greater emphasis on mutuality and social solidarity (Saltman and Figueras 1998; Wynand and Schut 2008). European health insurance-based systems have been generically typified as 'corporatist' or 'conservative-corporatist' (Dent 2003b; Esping-Andersen 1990; Wendt et al 2009) and were later adopters of NPM than the tax based systems of the UK, Scandinavia and Southern Europe. This tended, as one would expect, to also delay the reorganisation of health and social services and impact on the professionals involved. Indeed, Germany proved to be the most resistant to this rationalising managerial movement, but eventually it too adopted its own version (Dent 2005).

However, our health and social care systems in the UK have evolved beyond the basic NPM model outlined earlier. Nevertheless, most of the criteria (Hood 1991, 1995) are now well embedded in the organisation and delivery of these services. The one partial exception has been the expectation that 'managerialism' would replace 'professional dominance', whereas in reality the issue of 'dominance' whether by managers or professionals has been transmogrified and embedded within a newer narrative of leadership (Currie and Lockett 2011). But before this is examined further, we need to look at the impact the NPM had on health and social care that led to the growth of support work in hospitals, care homes and other parallel settings.

The rise of support workers in nursing

Care workers, otherwise known as health and social care support workers, are predominantly women who provide the bulk of hands-on care in hospitals and care homes. In the UK, and especially within the English systems of social and health care delivery, the main driver for the creation of the modern generation of health care support workers was the further professionalisation of nurses, in a manner that fits well into a neo-Weberian analysis of social closure. It was initiated with the policy of Project 2000 (Bowman 1995; UKCC 1986). Part of the intention was to develop a stronger scientific and philosophical basis to nursing care, which was seen to necessitate changes to the system of nurse education and training (Walby et al 1994). This marked a clear move towards nursing becoming a graduate profession, but it would appear to have also been a Faustian pact with the state, for in return for increased opportunities for professional specialisation and status, it was accepted that many of the traditional routine, but more caring, nursing tasks would be carried out by a new (or revamped) body of less qualified and lower paid workers – health care assistants (HCAs). Moreover, this 'new' body of health care workers would be more directly under the control of management than nursing (Kessler et al 2010). They are, equally, part of the nursing team in terms of task allocation, although there are issues over role boundaries and lines of responsibility (Cavendish 2013).

Within the hospital setting, the 1990 NHS and Community Care Act introduced the grade of HCA, and did so explicitly as a replacement for student nurses following the implementation of Project 2000 – as the related reforms to nursing education and training meant student nurses had become supernumerary on the wards. The Act also marked a shift in emphasis in the care of the elderly from the public to the private/independent sector. This provided a very different work environment for health care support workers than their opposite numbers in social care (Cavendish 2013). Those health support staff working as nursing auxiliaries had long been in existence, but the changes brought about following the NHS and Community Care Act reflected an NPM agenda. This was because of its focus on rejigging the mix of skills and staffing in order to be able to utilise more extensively lower paid support workers, including HCAs, relative to the numbers of skilled professionals. In social care, principally in nursing homes, the managerialist drive was compounded further by the policy of contracting care in the private sector, which also had a similar impact, with the consequence that the sector is challenged with problems of staff retention (Cavendish 2013; Skills for Care 2018). By way of comparison, a similar trend can be identified within Swedish nursing homes, which historically were even more professionally dominated that in the UK. These have also been redefined as *social services*-oriented activities as distinct from *medically*-oriented roles as in previous times (Hasselbladh and Selander 2003), thereby indicating a line of potential convergence between the two countries.

Within the hospital sector by contrast, the UK government promoted nursing's own bid for greater professional expertise and status. This was not a reflection of any substantive recognition of the claims of the profession, but driven more by the same NPM logic as that applying to support workers. This was because the new 'skill mix' arrangements meant suitably trained and qualified nurses could now substitute for doctors to a greater extent than ever before (Dent 2003b). The move also created a space for the expansion and remodelling of nursing auxiliaries work. But before this point is expanded, more needs to be said on related nursing developments across Europe.

Here there have been similar changes where the education of first level nurses also moved into higher education. The process, though, has been slow, with nurses in several countries continuing to qualify through nursing schools attached to hospitals, including in France and Germany (Robinson and Griffiths 2007) and Italy (Dent 2002). Indeed, even where there were nursing departments within universities – as in Greece – the nursing profession had long been up against a widespread public perception that nursing was of low status compared to other health professions. This has in part been because of the assumption that nurses are people who were not intelligent enough to qualify for a higher status health profession, like medicine (Dent 2003b). A consequence of this is that it is unlikely there will be any expansion of institutional support work, including through HCAs. This is also related to the already mentioned tradition of 'familialism' (Dent 2003a; Marí-Klose and Moreno-Fuentes 2013; Trifiletti 1999) that dictates that the family provides the caring work for their sick or frail elderly relatives. From the professionalisation of nursing perspective, the situation is further exacerbated by the over production of doctors (Dent 2002) with the consequence that they continue to carry out tasks long since absorbed within nursing in Northern European countries, leaving little space for nursing to develop more scientifically and philosophically.

The case of social work and social care education and training has been even more mixed, in that the routinisation of procedures in the wake of neo-liberal NPM policies (Carey 2008; Garrett 2010) has not been ameliorated by any professional upgrading as in the case of nursing. But here the nature of social care in institutional settings has been characterised much more by privatisation (Scourfield 2007) and a large expansion in support workers relative to social care and nursing professional staff (Carey 2008). Overall in the UK the number of full-time equivalent support worker jobs are estimated at 1.13 million, with the number of people working full and part time in adult social care judged to be around 1.47 million, of which some 1.35 million jobs are in the independent sector (78 per cent) and the local authority sector (7 per cent) combined. The remainder such as HCAs are either employed in the NHS or external institutional care (Skills for Care 2018). This is partly because, as Cavendish (2013) points out, it is not compulsory for employers to regularly report their workforce figures coupled with the high turnover rate within this group, which currently runs at over 30 per cent (Skills for Care 2018).

Nursing professionalisation and support workers

The problem for nurse professionalisation has long been the ambivalent relationship between nursing as *care work* and nursing as *clinical work*. In attempting to solve this tension with the implementation of Project 2000, nursing in the UK may well have benefitted professionally from the impact of the NPM. This is because it provided the logic that created the revamped workforce of support staff within both clinical and care home settings and created greater opportunities for specialist and consultant nurse roles. Even so, there is still the lingering suggestion within some organisational and sociological analyses that nursing is a semi-profession (Katz 1969; Muzio et al 2019) as it includes the emotional labour and/or sentimental work of patient care (Smith 2012). The mistake here is that the semi-professionalism argument wrongly assumes that nursing in contemporary health care organisations does not require any degree of theoretical knowledge or managerial acumen and is always and necessarily subordinate to medical jurisdiction. These assumptions fail to account for the recent changes to nursing and medicine's institutional relations with the state in the UK and elsewhere. They came about as a response to calls for greater accountability and demands for greater efficiencies, which have also been important in the rationalisation of the management of support workers, particularly within the health sector.

Support workers, by contrast, whether in social care or the health sector, are not professionals in any organised, institutionalised sense. As this volume indicates throughout, this is indeed one of the defining features of such work. Nonetheless, in relation to nursing, given that many patients and their family and friends tend to assume all the staff in nursing-style uniform on the hospital ward are nurses, the statement warrants some scrutiny. There are other relevant and important reasons for giving the issue of professional status closer examination too. First, much of the work HCAs carry out was once done by registered nurses. Second, the work of HCAs – if not all care workers – now falls within the professional jurisdiction and direction of nursing. Third, the work of these staff is largely governed by professional protocols with the expectation they will be followed in a spirit of professionalism. I am not here making a case for the professionalisation of support workers, but rather providing a lens on the changing nature of professions and professionalism. This section will examine the implications of these three points in relation to the interconnections between the profession of nursing and support workers in social and health care.

The professional project in its various historical forms (Johnson 2016; Larson 1977; Macdonald 1995), whether interpreted through a neo-Weberian or a neo-Marxian perspective, has been a masculine construction, or as Witz (1992:3) pithily put it, 'professional men's own construction of their gendered self-image'. This is highly relevant to the professionalisation project of nursing (Dent 2003b) and by association the expansion of the support workforce as both groups are predominantly female. It would be too much of a detour here to revisit the professionalisation strategy of British nursing (see Witz 1992; Davies 1995). Nevertheless, it is necessary to emphasise some key points drawing on a neo-Weberian perspective to make sense of the current professionalism narrative vis-à-vis support workers. As with several other aspirational occupations, including schoolteachers and social workers, nurses from the second half of the 19th century onwards actively sought formal professional recognition, autonomy and status. On a day-to-day basis nurses worked alongside medical men and were largely considered the 'doctors' handmaidens' (in a gendered way as the phrase implies). They were particularly challenged by the force of patriarchy in their aim to seek professional status and their own jurisdiction independent of medicine. Nurses were concerned to win self-governance and overall control of their occupation – underpinned by legislation, representing *heteronomous control*. They also needed to try and ensure their medical colleagues were forced to recognise nursing's own jurisdiction and autonomy independent of their own. In other words, nurses were fighting on two fronts: to gain professional status and autonomy by legislative means; and to gain professional independence from the jurisdictional power the medical profession over their work. Nurses were never wholly satisfied with the professional settlement gained within the 1919 Nurse Registration Act, although the implementation of the later Briggs (1972) report, and more especially Project 2000 in the 1990s (Macdonald 1995), did somewhat redress the sense of professional grievance. It was Project 2000 that led to the notion that nursing for nurses was becoming a genuinely professional occupation.

This professional agenda had a very direct impact on the expansion of support work in both health and social care, a link that illustrated the interplay between professionalisation and the NPM. Initially, the expansion of the use of support workers in the wake of Project 2000 was a cost control strategy, since it provided a cheaper alternative to nurses, as well as other allied professionals. Support workers took on the routine and less skilled tasks (as, for instance, assisting with the feeding and toileting of old and frail patients). But, with time, this also extended to include more skilled work, including catheterisation and taking venous blood samples (Cavendish 2013). While the policy within hospitals can be understood in terms of the consequence of the new nurse professionalisation related to Project 2000, its impact was far less obvious in the community. There, while nurse professionalisation was relevant, it was more significant that care and residential homes were being increasingly privatised, which reflected more strongly the marketisation logic of the NPM. These two forces of privatisation and professionalisation were also reflected in the managerial discourse on 'skill mix' in the delivery of care. The concept is designed to ensure the high cost of professional work is minimised by substituting qualified nurses with unqualified and lower paid support workers wherever possible in order to control costs (Cavendish 2013). Overall, the aim is to provide as good a quality of patient and client care in times of diminishing resources and demographically driven growing demand – and need – for health and social care. In the reshaping of the professions – with nursing taking on clinical tasks previously carried out solely by physicians – the space within the division of labour for 'hands-on' patient and client care grew and was further expanded by the growing demand from a longer living population. This care work has now largely been designated as support work within health and social care.

This new division of nursing-type labour was one that was not uncontested. While the reforms of the nursing profession across Europe towards the latter end of the 20th century were meant to give nurses a sense of having achieved greater professionalisation, many within the profession were worried that something important was being lost in taking on more clinical responsibilities as nurse specialists, nurse consultants and related roles. There was a real sense that a key component of nursing was disappearing, that of patient/client care (Dent and Burtney 1997) – that is, the time to treat patients holistically, including elements of 'hands-on' care, and all in order to provide an economically efficient skill mix. That was the key principle although the picture in the UK has been a little more complex. By 2013, when Cavendish reported, there were wide variations across the sectors with no clear boundaries between the work of some HCAs and that of nurses, nor any standardisation across the service in relation to the grading of HCAs. There were basically three grades, with the great majority of HCAs designated as Band 2 (Cavendish 2013). More recently, a new higher grade of Band 4 Assistant Practitioner (AP) has been introduced. These APs are tasked with carrying out work previously undertaken by nurses under their jurisdiction. This was also intended to help provide a career structure for HCAs, and a pathway into the nursing profession, especially for those recruits who preferred an apprenticeship route into nursing (Cavendish 2013). This points to a new dynamic both in managerialism and professionalism. For support workers working in care homes pay and status have been less attractive relative to those within the NHS, a situation not helped by the fragmented organisation of the sector. To illustrate this, the Competition and Markets Authority (2017) reported that:

> there are around 5,500 different providers in the UK operating 11,300 care homes for the elderly. Around 95% of their beds are provided by the independent sector (both for-profit and charitable providers) ... [Local Authorities] generally commission care services from independent care providers.

And while homes are regulated by the Care Quality Commission (https://cqc.org.uk), the opportunities and conditions for support workers in this sector compare unfavourably with their colleagues within the health sector. Within the health and social care sector, initially the generic support workforce became the non-professional and formally unskilled body of workers that provided personal patient and client care. There was some ambiguity as to whether they were support workers for the nurses or the patients/clients. In hospitals the expectation was that the management of the HCAs was the nurses' responsibility. Another development has been the tendency for some HCAs to 'work above their grade' and be tasked with 'taking bloods' and other similar clinical procedures. In this connection there was even a call for support workers to be more accountable and to be registered by the Professional Standards Authority for Health and Social Care (Allsop and Jones 2018; PSA 2016; Saks and Allsop 2007). The crucial point here is that any registration process was not intended to formalise the support workers' jurisdiction, whether working in hospitals or care homes, but instead to enable their better management and supervision (Saks and Allsop 2007).

While the nursing profession has undergone changes that ostensibly reinforce professional status, a parallel process has impacted on support work, including that of HCAs, which is not a process of professionalisation, but something akin to 'responsibilisation' (Fournier 1999). In other words, this workforce is expected to be strongly motivated by professional-type values, notably client and patient care of a high standard, coupled with a ready willingness to take direct responsibility for the delivery of such care. Yet, support workers formally do not have any significant levels of autonomy or discretion, nor any professional associations. Instead, they are arguably a proto-professional workforce (Dent and Pahor 2015) who work largely within the auspices of the jurisdiction of the health professions and are familiar with the language and culture of the health professions, but are not part of it. Before developing this theme further, however, it is necessary to explain more about the trajectory of health and social care management and leadership – which has seen an increasing transition from the NPM to the NPG – to bring this account more up-to-date.

From the New Public Management to the New Public Governance

In the UK the report by Francis (2013) was a particularly important and critical inquiry into the real and often inhumane shortcomings of a highly managerialised system of delivering hospital care and has also gone on to have a major influence on social care. As has been seen, the inquiry led on to a much shorter report by Cavendish (2013) on the work and management of health and social care support workers. This latter review identified the main concerns associated with organisation and delivery of support work within health and social care settings, and recommended a clear policy that in organisational terms marked a moving on from the NPM towards more of an NPG approach, even if that specific terminology was not directly used.

The new arrangements in the health and social care sectors were not without their consequences. In part this reflected growing pressure of demand on both sectors and concerns over the limitations on funding, especially within social care (Bottery et al 2019). The situation would have been even more difficult financially had the substitution of support workers for skilled nurses in health and social care not happened. There was another important element to the new managerialism particularly relevant within the health sector – the emphasis on performance targets. These targets marked a relentless drive for greater efficiency and, in connection with the support worker labour force, including HCAs, led to concerns of overwork, inadequate supervision and training as they often were the only effective human resource available to deliver care *qua* care to clients and patients (Cavendish 2013). This marked the beginnings of a shift in emphasis away from *management* and more towards *leadership* (Currie and Lockett 2011).

Some 20 or more years after the NPM had reshaped support work, along with nursing and care work more generally, moves could be discerned to introduce reforms that began to mitigate the weaknesses in the quality of care it provided. In part this was related to identifying clearly who was responsible for the management and leadership of support workers, but what emerged at a practical level was a greater emphasis on governance. While this shifted more attention on to the specifics of governance, it created space for greater leadership relative to management within the service. There was therefore considerable focus on transformational leadership as the way forward, even if what appears to have taken root is something more akin to distributed leadership (Currie and Lockett 2011) facilitated within a system of care pathways and clinical governance guidelines. There are two caveats to this perspective. The first is that, in order to for the sector to move from the NPM to the NPG in the form of guidelines and pathways, this might itself be reasonably viewed as 'transformational', albeit reflecting the increasing influence of health professionals within a contested terrain of health and social care. The second caveat is that – despite devolution to constituent countries – the NHS within the UK is highly centralised and politicised, which may make it impossible to move to a distributed leadership model, even though the complexity of health and social services is such that neither detailed centralised management nor 'heroic' transformational leadership is likely to be able to provide sustained system stability.

The evolving alternative narrative to the NPM which has been referred to as the NPG (Newman 2001; Osborne 2006, 2010) has gained traction within the past 20 years. In its optimistic version it was viewed as a system that would guarantee good quality services based on networks and mutuality (Ferlie 2012). In reality, and in the context of reduced public spending, the NPG was less of a rejection of managerialism and more a realisation of its growing limitations. This meant, instead of pushing for greater managerial controls on health care professionals and health and social care support workers, a new system of 'self-management' was set up. The discourse changed from 'management' to 'leadership' partly no doubt because this would appeal more to the nursing and medical staff that were being recruited into managerial-type roles. This development has been much analysed in terms of 'hybrids' and the question of whether one could be both a transactional manager and a values-driven professional (Dent and Bode 2014; Dent et al 2012; Noordegraaf 2015). Here it is useful to read the discourse of O'Reilly and Reed (2012:37) on 'leaderism', a more cynical take on the current interest in leadership within UK public services that attempts to reconcile 'a broad and complex spectrum of cultural values and organizational practices'.

The new leadership approach was to be achieved for support workers in health and social care by shifting recruitment and training much more towards a values-driven approach – with the focus on 'caring' rather than efficiency (Cavendish 2013) and this was reflected in a new body of regulations registered with the Professional Standards Authority for Health and Social Care (Allsop and Jones 2018). This would appear to give the support workers a *prima facie* professional status and casts new light on the old, and now widely rejected, concept of semi-professionalism mentioned earlier (Katz 1969). This parallels the same Janus-faced trend that that is driving the related current wave of user and patient involvement within the sector (O'Reilly and Reed 2012). It seems to be 'empowering' the patients and users in the latter case (Dent and Pahor 2015) and in the former case the support workers in health and social care themselves. The reality has been a system redesign that is more oriented to better deliver services within tight budgets against a backdrop of an expanding demographic demand for services. It is at the interface between the professionals and the users that we find health and social care workers attempting to 'square the circle' between what is required and what can actually be delivered. These support workers, in combination with their professional colleagues, provide the 'loose coupling' (Weick 1976) or 'de-coupling' (Meyer and Rowan 1991), whereby formal organisational rules are interpreted creatively to get the work completed more effectively. Both are illuminating concepts in making sense of how care is actually delivered and commonly known as 'work arounds' (Dent and Tutt 2014). If done well, this involves an accurate, but flexible interpretation of the client or patient's needs. This connects with a particularity of such work – namely, that it usually involves an element of emotional labour (Smith 2012). Moreover, it is also largely gendered as women's work since 84 per cent of support staff are female (Cavendish 2013), with related assumptions of tacit skills (Kessler, Heron and Dopson 2015).

Support workers, professionalism and responsibilisation

Finally, let us return to the issue of professionalism, but this time in light of the preceding discussion on the NPG and leadership. While it may seem a circuitous route, we start with the medical profession. The physicians' own clinical autonomy has shifted significantly away from the individual physician and has become a more collective autonomy shared within the professional group. The vehicles for this shift include the growing use of medical protocols – or guidelines. These are intended to integrate into the multidisciplinary care pathways that bring together not only medical and surgical specialities, but also nursing, support workers, patients, carers and others besides (Allen 2009; Dent and Tutt 2014). The logic of integrating care around these pathways is currently redefining the provision of health care and often redefining patients' routes through the health and social care systems. These are intended to underpin the delivery of high-quality care and embody agreed 'best practice'. The design and implementation of care pathways are meant to be multidisciplinary and all contributors – whether doctors, nurses, support workers, patients or clients – are expected to follow them, although there is some variation as to how the various work groups/professions interpret this (Allen 2014).

Care guidelines and pathways shape the work of the support workers, including HCAs and, as such, provide the framework for delivering 'professional' patient-centred care. It reflects the shift from the NPM to the NPG, from an overt 'labour process' managerialism to an embedded system of governance. In other words, rather than checking retrospectively whether the work has been carried out to the required level of efficiency and quality, this is programmed into the guidelines. The system contains the essentials of Foucault's 'governmentality' or Latour's 'action at a distance' (Miller and Rose 2008) – in other words, the management of the work processes is plumbed into the guidelines that are contained in the care pathways. The other important point is that, unlike the NPM, this newer arrangement incorporates more directly professional, evidence-based, criteria. This means in turn that support workers, in so far as they follow the guidelines in a committed way, exhibit a form of 'proto-professionalism', in which their actions and talk emulate the work of their professional colleagues, but are not grounded in the training, socialisation or responsibility associated with full professionalism. Medical and nursing students go through a similar proto-professionalism stage on their journey to becoming fully qualified professionals (Dent and Pahor 2015). As noted earlier, this adoption of a quasi-professional approach to work can also be referred to as 'responsibilisation' (Fournier 1999) which, in this instance, relates to the expectation that support workers will behave in more of a 'values-driven' professional way – while not being members of an organised profession themselves.

Conclusion

What is especially fascinating about the growth and development of support workers in the health and social care sectors has been how they have shifted away from being simply support carers managed in a similar way to cleaners and porters. Instead, as particularly illustrated by the case of nursing and their auxiliaries, they are being increasingly seen as staff who are more effective when imbued with the sentiments of professionalism, even if they do not have the full, legally underpinned exclusionary social closure of a profession as defined in a neo-Weberian approach (Saks 2010). The initial policy driver had been to provide a cheaper substitute work for a higher paid, qualified nursing staff. This economistic approach, however, created its own problems. First, there was the question as to who managed the support workers. Second, there was the challenge of low morale and high labour turnover. Third, there were the implications for the quality of patient and client care. These are each now considered in turn by way of a conclusion.

As regards the first issue of management – and subsequently leadership too – initially the NPM was as much about putting managers in charge as it was about making organisations more efficient. However, the experience within the health services and any organisation with a predominantly professional workforce suggests that this is not possible at a practical level. Consequently, over time, health support workers have to some degree become part of nursing, and indeed other health professional team, and managed within the professional frame. This was further reinforced with the shift in emphasis within health care organisations towards systems governance designed to create clinical and other pathways under the NPG. Where the approach has been slower to develop, as in social care, there has tended to be lower work morale and high labour turnover. Although this issue is more complex than simply a change of leadership style, unless there is such a commitment within the organisation, support workers may not be positively engaged with their work, nor their patients and clients. This then has consequences for the third issue – namely, that of the quality of patient and client care. Only as adjuncts to health professions such as nursing and providing 'hands-on' care within professional jurisdictions can it reasonably be supposed that good quality care can be maintained. It is this group of support workers that comes closest to the concept of the 'semi-professional' in the sense of being a non-professional group working within a professional jurisdiction. This is further accentuated with the relatively recent extension of the career grades beyond the HCA to include the AP, which can provide an entry into the health profession itself. In this sense, this category of support worker may be more 'proto-professional' than 'semi-professional' in the strict definition of these terms – in its specific location as first a managed and now an increasingly led resource within the health care division of labour.

References

Allen, D. (2009) 'From boundary concept to boundary object: The practice and politics of care pathway development', *Social Science and Medicine* 69: 354–61.

Allen, D. (2014) 'Lost in translation? "Evidence" and the articulation of institutional logics in integrated care pathways: From positive to negative boundary object?', *Sociology of Health and Illness* 36(6): 808–22.

Allsop, J. and Jones, K. (2018) 'Regulating the regulators: The rise of the United Kingdom Professional Standards Authority', in Chamberlain, J.M., Dent, M. and Saks, M. (eds) *Professional Health Regulation in the Public Interest: International Perspectives*, Bristol: Policy Press.

Bottery, S., Ward, D. and Fenney, D. (2019) 'Social Care 360', www.kingsfund.org.uk/publications/social-care-360

Bowman M. (1995) *The Professional Nurse*, Boston, MA: Springer.

Briggs, A. (1972) *Report of the Committee on Nursing*, London: HMSO.

Carey, M. (2008) 'Everything must go? The privatisation of state social work', *British Journal of Social Work* 38: 918–35.

Cavendish, C. (2013) *An Independent Review into Healthcare Assistants and Support Workers in the NHS and Social Care Settings*, https://assets. publishing.service.gov.uk/government/uploads/system/uploads/ attachment_data/file/236212/Cavendish_Review.pdf

Christensen, T. and Laegreid, P. (2011) *The Ashgate Companion to New Public Management*, Farnham: Ashgate.

Competition and Markets Authority (2017) *Care Homes Market Study: Summary of Final Report*, www.gov.uk/government/publications/ care-homes-market-study-summary-of-final-report/care-homes- market-study-summary-of-final-report

Currie, G. and Lockett, A. (2011) 'Distributing leadership in health and social care: Concertive, conjoint or collective?', *International Journal of Management Reviews* 13: 286–300.

Davies, C. (1995) *Gender and the Professional Predicament in Nursing*, Buckingham: Open University Press.

Dent, M. (2002) 'Professional predicaments: Comparing the professionalisation projects of German and Italian nurses', *International Journal of Public Sector Management* 15(2): 151–62.

Dent, M. (2003a) 'Nurse professionalisation and traditional values in Poland and Greece', *International Journal of Public Sector Management* 16(2): 153–62.

Dent, M. (2003b) *Remodelling Hospitals and Health Professions in Europe: Medicine, Nursing and the State*, Basingstoke: Palgrave Macmillan.

Dent, M. (2005) 'Post-new public management in public sector hospitals? The UK, Germany and Italy', *Policy and Politics* 33(4): 623–36.

Dent, M. (2015) 'Professions and managers', in Wilkinson, A., Townsend, K. and Suder, G. (eds) *Handbook of Research on Managing Managers*, Cheltenham: Edward Elgar.

Dent, M. and Burtney, E. (1997) 'Changes in practice nursing: Professionalism, segmentation and sponsorship', *Journal of Clinical Nursing* 6: 355–63.

Dent, M. and Bode, I. (2014) 'Introduction: Converging hybrid worlds? Medicine and hospital management in Europe', *International Journal of Public Sector Management* 27(5), https://doi.org/10.1108/ IJPSM-01-2013-0011

Dent, M., Kirkpatrick, I. and Neogy, I. (2012) 'Medical leadership and management reforms in hospital: A comparative study', in Teelken, C., Ferlie, E. and Dent, M. (eds) *Leadership in the Public Sector: Promises and Pitfalls*, London: Routledge.

Dent, M. and Pahor, M. (2015) 'Patient involvement in Europe: A comparative perspective', *Journal of Health Organization and Management* 29(5): 546–55.

Dent, M. and Tutt, D. (2014) 'Electronic patient information systems and care pathways: The organisational challenges of implementation and integration', *Health Informatics Journal* 20(3): 176–88.

Esping-Andersen, G. (1990) *The Three Worlds of Welfare Capitalism*, Cambridge: Polity Press.

Ferlie, E. (2012) 'Concluding discussion: Paradigms and instruments of public management reform – the question of agency', in Teelken, C., Ferlie, E. and Dent, M. (eds) *Leadership in the Public Sector: Promises and Pitfalls*, London: Routledge.

Fournier, V. (1999) 'The appeal of "professionalism" as a disciplinary mechanism', *Sociological Review* 47(2): 280–307.

Francis, R. (2013) *Report of the Mid Staffordshire NHS Foundation Trust Public Inquiry*, London: The Stationery Office, www.gov.uk/government/publications/report-of-the-mid-staffordshire-nhs-foundation-trust-public-inquiry

Garrett, P.M. (2010) 'Examining the "conservative revolution": Neoliberalism and social work education', *Social Work Education* 29(4): 340–55.

Hasselbladh, H. and Selander, M. (2003) 'Plural frames of work in public sector organisations', in Barry, J.M., Dent, M. and O'Neill, M. (eds) *Gender and the Public Sector: Professionals and Managerial Change*, London: Routledge.

Hood, C. (1991) 'A public management for all seasons?', *Public Administration* 69: 3–19.

Hood, C. (1995) 'The "New Public Management" in the 1980s: Variations on a theme', *Accounting, Organizations and Society* 20(2–3): 93–109.

Jeffries, M., Mathieson, A., Kennedy, A., Kirk, S., Morris, R., Blickem, C., Vassilev, I. and Rogers, A. (2015) 'Participation in voluntary and community organisations in the UK and the influences on the self-management of long-term conditions', *Health and Social Care in the Community* 23(3): 252–61.

Johnson, T.J. (2016) *Professions and Power*, Abingdon: Routledge Revivals.

Katz, F.E. (1969) 'Nurses', in Etzioni, A. (ed) *The Semi-Professions and their Organizations: Teachers, Nurses, Social Workers*, New York: The Free Press.

Kessler, I., Heron, P. and Dopson, S. (2015) 'Managing patient emotions as skilled work and being "one of us"', *Work, Employment and Society* 39(5): 775–91.

Kessler, I., Heron, P., Dopson, S., Magee, H. and Swain, D. (2010) *Nature and Consequences of Support Workers in a Hospital Setting. Final Report*, London: NIHR Service Delivery and Organisation programme.

Kirkpatrick, I. (2006) 'Between markets and networks: The reform of social care provision in the UK', *Revista de Análisis Económico* 21(2): 43–59, http://ssrn.com/abstract=1241003

Klein, R. (2013) *The New Politics of the NHS: From Creation to Reinvention*, 7th edition, Abingdon: Radcliffe Publishing.

Larson, M.S. (1977) *The Rise of Professionalism: A Sociological Analysis*, Berkeley, CA: University of California Press.

Macdonald, K.M. (1995) *The Sociology of the Professions*, London: Sage.

Marí-Klose, P. and Moreno-Fuentes, F.J. (2013) 'The Southern European welfare model in the post-industrial order: Still a distinctive cluster?', *Journal European Societies* 15(4): 475–92.

Meyer, J.W. and Rowan, B. (1991) 'Institutional organizations: Formal structure as myth and ceremony', in Powell W.W. and DiMaggio, P.J. (eds) *The New Institutionalism in Organizational Analysis*, Chicago, IL: University of Chicago Press.

Miller, P. and Rose, N. (2008) *Governing the Present*, Cambridge: Polity Press.

Milligan, C. (2018) *Geographies of Care: Space, Place and the Voluntary Sector*, London: Routledge.

Muzio, D., Aulakh, S. and Kirkpatrick, I. (2019) *Professional Occupations and Organizations* (Elements of Organizational Theory e-book series), Cambridge: Cambridge University Press.

Newman, J. (2001) *Modernising Governance*, London: Sage.

Noordegraaf, M. (2015) 'Hybrid professionalism and beyond: (New) Forms of public professionalism in changing organizational and societal contexts', *Journal of Professions and Organization* 2: 187–206.

O'Reilly, D. and Reed, M. (2012) '"Leaderism" and the discourse of leadership in the reformation of UK public services', in Teelken, C., Ferlie, E. and Dent, M. (eds) *Leadership in the Public Sector: Promises and Pitfalls*, London: Routledge.

Osborne, S. (2006) 'The new public governance', *Public Management Review* 8(3): 377–87.

Osborne, S. (2010) *The New Public Governance?* London: Routledge.

Pollitt, C. and Bouckaert, G. (2011) *Public Management Reform: A Comparative Analysis*, Oxford: Oxford University Press.

Pollock, A.M. (2005) *NHS plc: The Privatisation of Our Health Care*, London: Verso.

PSA (2016) *Regulation Rethought*, London: Professional Standards Authority.

Robinson, S. and Griffiths, P. (2007) *Nursing Education and Regulation: International Profiles and Perspectives*, Kings College London, https://eprints.soton.ac.uk/348772/1/NurseEduProfiles.pdf

Robinson, R., Gregory, S. and Jabbal, J. (2014) *The Social Care and Health Systems of Nine Countries*, London: The King's Fund, www.kingsfund.org.uk/sites/default/files/media/commission-background-paper-social-care-health-system-other-countries.pdf

Saks, M. (2010) 'Analyzing the professions: The case for a neo-Weberian approach', *Comparative Sociology* 9(6): 887–915.

Saks, M. and Allsop, J. (2007) 'Social policy, professional regulation and health support work in the UK', *Social Policy and Society* 6(2):165–77.

Saltman, R.B. and Figueras, J. (1998) 'The evidence on European health care reforms', *Health Affairs*, 17(2), https://doi.org/10.1377/hlthaff.17.2.85

Scourfield, P. (2007) 'Are there reasons to be worried about the "caretelisation" of residential care?', *Critical Social Policy* 27(2): 155–81.

Skills for Care (2018) *The State of the Adult Social Care Sector and Workforce in England*, www.skillsforcare.org.uk/NMDS-SC-intelligence/Workforce-intelligence/documents/State-of-the-adult-social-care-sector/The-state-of-the-adult-social-care-sector-and-workforce-2018.pdf

Smith, P. (2012) *The Emotional Labour of Nursing Revisited: Can Nurses Still Care?* 2nd edition, Basingstoke: Palgrave Macmillan.

Trifiletti, R. (1999) 'Southern European welfare regimes and the worsening position of women', *Journal of European Social Policy* 9(1): 49–64.

UKCC (1986) *Project 2000: A New Perspective for Practice*, London: United Kingdom Central Council for Nursing, Midwifery and Health Visiting.

Walby, S., Greenwell, J., Mackay, L. and Soothill, K. (1994) *Medicine and Nursing: Professions in a Changing Health Service*, London: Sage.

Weick, K.E. (1976) 'Educational organizations as loosely coupled systems', *Administrative Science Quarterly* 21: 1–19.

Wendt, C., Frisina, L. and Rothgang, H. (2009) 'Healthcare system types: A conceptual framework for comparison', *Social Policy and Administration* 43(1): 70–90.

Wilsford, D. (1994) 'Path dependency, or why history makes it difficult but not impossible to reform health care systems in a big way', *Journal of Public Policy* 14(3): 251–83.

Witz, A. (1992) *Professions and Patriarchy*, London: Routledge.

Wynand, P.M.M. and Schut, F.T. (2008) 'Universal mandatory health insurance in The Netherlands: A model of the United States?', *Health Affairs* 27(3), https://doi.org/10.1377/hlthaff.27.3.771

FIVE

Regulation, risk and health support work

Mike Saks and Judith Allsop

Introduction: health professionalisation, risk and the public interest

This chapter discusses the limited regulation and management of risk in the work of support workers in health and social care compared to the more rigorous regulation of health professionals. It is evident that health care systems in the modern world are increasingly dependent on such workers. This is in part due to growing demand from ageing populations with multiple health and social care needs that require a mix of skills to provide care, but also to shortages in the supply, and the cost of, highly trained professionals (McKee et al 2006). Here, a neo-Weberian perspective has been adopted to analyse the role of professional groups in the health care division of labour. The focus is on the UK and particularly on England as policies now differ from Northern Ireland, Scotland and Wales. This perspective takes the stance that professions have gained exclusionary social closure over particular areas of work, underwritten by the state in a competitive marketplace (Saks 2010). Such closure has involved the establishment of registers on which appear the names of a limited group of those eligible, who typically have the requisite graduate level educational credentials and are subject to ethical codes and mechanisms of disciplinary enforcement. This has allowed the development of policies for the regulation and management of risk. By comparison, health support workers, a large and heterogeneous group, are less subject to entry requirements and regulatory oversight. As highlighted in various chapters of this book, this is the case in a number of other modern countries.

For the health professions, self-regulatory, monopolistic arrangements have been the norm. This form of regulation has been theorised in different ways. For example, functionalist writers have seen self-regulation as in the public interest, in which a profession regulates specialised expertise of great value to society on behalf of the state.

In this arrangement, a monopoly to practise is gained as a trade-off and the profession is collectively rewarded by enhanced income, status and power (Goode 1960). Later theorists of the professions have viewed this as part of the occupational rhetoric of professionalism. Thus, Marxist writers tend to see the health and other professions as maintaining and extending their position by acting as agents of control and surveillance for the dominant capitalist class (Esland 1980), while Foucauldians challenge the progressive image of professions by highlighting their role in harness with the state as an extension of the process of governmentality (Johnson 1995). Neo-Weberians argue that the apparent protection of the public against risk offered by the altruistic ideologies of professions can be subverted by their group self-interests. However, neither this nor the other theoretical positions outlined are always underpinned by a strong evidence base (Saks 2016b).

Despite these theoretical differences, it is clear that health work as an area of practice has become of increasing significance in the modern state. Technological developments and rising public demand have elevated awareness of the gap between good and poor practice and the presence of risk to patient safety in interventions to secure good health. In consequence, public policy has focused on minimising risk. Beck (1992) has argued that we live in a 'risk society' in an increasingly uncertain world with many seismic environmental, technological and other challenges, even if some authors suggest that risks have been overestimated (see Burgess 2016). Nevertheless, successive governments in the UK and elsewhere have made significant efforts both in their policy narrative and policy changes to mitigate risk through increased professional regulation, particularly with regard to the medical profession (Saks 2016a). As Alaszewski (2016) comments, the concept of risk underpins the current relationship between health experts and citizens and is central to the system of modern health care. There is therefore greater reliance on mechanisms such as audit and the wider use of evidence-based protocols by health professionals to assure quality and safety.

Risks vary according to the work context. In this chapter, we aim to consider the policy developments in managing risk in the client and wider public interest among health professions and associated occupations, including health support workers. We will argue that certain professions are highly regulated because risks have been well documented, while for others less is known about the incidence of risk. In the case of health support workers, there has been very little research on the risks involved. We know that work settings are diverse, tasks are variable, clients and patients tend to be vulnerable and a range of both paid and unpaid carers can be involved in a single case.

However, we do not know precisely the level, type and incidence of risk across different environments, although more is known about risks in institutional than in domestic settings. We will show that more health occupations are now subject to some form of regulation with a shift from a sharp divide between statutory professional regulation and non-regulation towards a greater variation in types of regulation.

The rise of risk-based regulation: adverse events and the policy response

In the UK relatively recent adverse events have led to the rise of a risk-based approach to health and social care governance with the development of protocols to guide decision making. For well over a decade the response of governments has been to set up inquiries followed by institutional changes and policies to oversee those working in health and social care settings. The aim has been to improve service quality and promote patient safety. This has changed the self-regulatory health professional landscape put in place from the mid-19th century. The key events over the past two decades are well known. In 2004 in the wake of the inquiry into the high rates of child mortality following paediatric surgery at the Bristol Royal Infirmary, the Council for Health Regulatory Excellence (CHRE) was established with a brief to oversee the nine health care professions regulated by statute, including doctors, dentists, nurses and pharmacists. This oversight body, linked to the Labour government's modernisation policy, was to extend regulation in the interests of public protection as a meta-regulator – in which regulatory processes were harmonised with greater accountability (Allsop and Saks 2002).

The shocking case of Dr Harold Shipman led to further reforms. Shipman, a general practitioner, was found to have murdered over 200 of his patients during a 30-year period without detection. The subsequent Inquiry chaired by Dame Janet Smith (2004) was followed by the Donaldson review of medical regulation (Department of Health 2006a) and the Foster review of the regulation of other health and social care professions (Department of Health 2006b). The pivotal White Paper *Trust, Assurance and Safety: The Regulation of Health Professionals in the 21st Century* (Department of Health 2007) linked to this case was incorporated through the 2008 Health and Social Care Act and resulted in a major restructuring of medicine and the health and care professions (Roche 2018). Other changes to protect the public have further transformed the medical profession from a self-regulated system to one that is now characterised by 'regulated self-regulation' (Chamberlain

2015). As part of this, regular appraisals have been instigated along with periodic reaccreditation procedures to ensure continuing fitness to practise. The adjudication of disciplinary cases through a tribunal with an independent legal chair has been introduced for the medical profession and is now gradually being rolled out more widely to other health professions. In 2012 the CHRE was renamed the Professional Standards Authority for Health and Social Care (PSA) and subsequently methods for annual scrutiny and monitoring were tightened with greater accountability of both the professional Councils and the meta-regulator subject to parliamentary scrutiny (Allsop and Jones 2018).

Other health professions in the UK also had their sentinel events that were heavily publicised in the media. These ranged from the murder and attempted murder of children in the case of nurse Beverley Allitt in Grantham (Askill and Sharpe 2014) to the poor standard of midwifery services in Morecambe Bay (Kirkup 2015). In social work, there was also the well-publicised case of 'Baby P', who was killed by his mother and stepfather despite the attentions of social workers and other health and care professionals (Jones 2014). The General Social Care Council had been established in 2001 to provide for the first time the professional regulation of social work. Its aim was to protect users, carers and the public. To this end, a Code of Practice was established for social care workers and employers in 2002, which was swiftly followed by a developing Social Care Register (General Social Care Council 2004). Qualified social workers along with social work students were registered shortly afterwards along with other types of social care workers, as the provisions were phased in. In terms of the risk to the public, this was mitigated to some degree through the encouragement given by the Council to abide by its Code of Practice alongside the Code for Employers, which covered the rights and interests of service users and was enforced by the National Care Standards Commission and Social Services Inspectorate (Saks and Allsop 2007). The Baby P case, however, led to the dissolution of the General Social Care Council in 2012 and the absorption of social work into the Health Professions Council, which henceforth became the Health and Care Professions Council (HCPC) (Saks 2015).

The HCPC is accountable to the PSA, which keeps a register of 16 health and social care occupations that governments have agreed to recognise as professions through statute – including, for example, biomedical scientists, practitioner psychologists and arts therapists, as well as social workers (Allsop and Jones 2018). These areas of work are based on professional expertise derived from training and qualifications, the practice of which carries an element of risk for users. A number of professions were registered in the early years. One such was operating department practitioners in 2004, a group that had previously been classified as non-professional health support workers (Saks et al 2000). In recent years, applications have only been accepted in exceptional circumstances, as shown by the recent rejection of applications from herbal practitioners and public health practitioners. Statutory professional regulation is sought as a mark of status, but also brings benefit for users through formal recognition of meeting governance criteria in terms of training and qualifications, maintaining standards of competence and having a procedure for dealing with complaints. Individual registrants can be warned, fined or ultimately barred from continuing to practise by being removed from the register in the interests of public protection.

Recent developments: an expansion of the regulatory gaze

Following the establishment of the PSA with its power to oversee, audit and appeal to the courts in relation to nine statutory Councils, there has been further stratification within the regulatory framework. We have already referred to the incorporation of new professions within the HCPC. Although this has virtually ceased in recent times, further developments have occurred in two directions: the expansion of associate professional roles overseen by Councils and the establishment of accredited occupations through the PSA. The PSA has gained the power to keep registers of the groups accredited by them, further extending the regulatory gaze in health and social care (Allsop and Jones 2018). These developments are now considered in turn.

Certain Councils regulate associate professionals – occupational groups working close to their general area of practice. For example, the General Medical Council regulates four groups of medical associates: associate physicians and associates in anaesthesia, surgery and advanced critical care. The General Dental Council oversees the practice of dental hygienists, dental nurses, dental technicians, and orthodontic therapists. The Nursing and Midwifery Council recognises associate professional nurses who work in a range of specific clinical support roles. They are referred to as assistant practitioners who may work independently although under the guidance of a fully qualified nurse across a variety of settings. The rationale for this division of labour is seen by the General Medical Council (2018) as a substitution of lower paid staff for highly trained professionals where there are shortages, thus containing or reducing the cost of health care services.

The extent of regulatory oversight of these groups extends from registration of competences and requirements for continuing professional development to supervision of task performance, although the new roles continue to develop. Some Councils, encouraged by state-level organisations, have devised career pathways for those in associate roles to progress through education and experience to more autonomous practice. The pay-off for such occupational groups is that they have a recognised area of expertise based on education and training and their practice is reviewed annually in a paper process to ensure continuing professional development by the Council responsible. It may be in the interests of professionals who employ associates to concentrate on specialised areas of practice, even if little is known about the benefits for associates – who may be employed part time in precarious work in various settings (see Chapter two). For those who use services, the plethora of titles and roles may be confusing and act as a barrier to understanding the expertise and level of training of those providing treatment and advice. The advantages or otherwise will depend on the management skills of employers at the local level.

In a further area of regulatory development, the PSA has gained powers to accredit health and care occupations and maintains a list of these. By 2015 there were 18 accredited registers covering 32 occupations recording almost 80,000 registrants (Professional Standards Authority 2015). Almost all of these related to what were termed 'talking or complementary' therapies and could be said to be subject to light regulation. The registers are voluntary, but registrants must meet certain governance criteria in terms of qualifications, be committed to following codes of practice and have a process for dealing with complaints. A quality mark, which must be renewed annually, is given to a registrant who meets the stated criteria for competence and trustworthiness. Those in such occupations can be struck off a register if they fail to reach the standards set and this may act as a barrier to entering another register. In sum, although associate professionals and accredited occupations have expanded the scope of regulation, the vast majority of those working in paid employment in the field of health and social care are not subject to such regulation. This chapter now considers the broader population of health support workers.

Health support workers: an understudied but risk-laden resource

In many countries, as previously suggested, a key cost-cutting strategy in face of rising public demand for services has been for agencies to substitute highly paid professionals for cheaper forms of labour through role enhancement, delegation and innovation (McKee et al 2006). Labour costs have long represented around two-thirds of overall health care costs in the NHS in the UK. As well as rising demand, other factors have introduced further constraints. For example, following the European Union working time directive, junior doctors' working hours had to be reduced, leading to rising costs (Klein 2013). The policy shift from hospitals to care in the community and the integration of health and social care also increased the demand for the recruitment of lower cost support workers (Ham 2009). Most of these health support workers are managed at the local level by health and social services or are employed by private sector organisations and/or the third sector. However, they have been neglected by researchers and policy makers alike despite being so numerous and vital to the wellbeing of the sick and vulnerable living in care institutions or receiving care in their own homes. It is notable that a government report entitled *A Health Service of All the Talents: Developing the NHS Workforce* (Department of Health 2000) entirely ignored paid health support workers – focusing instead solely on the professional labour force.

The risks associated with health support workers were very strikingly brought to the fore by the inquiry by Francis (2013). This provided evidence of the appallingly low standards of care at the Mid Staffordshire NHS Foundation Trust. Many, mostly elderly, patients within the Trust were found to have received poor care with low standards of hygiene being the norm, as well as there being serial instances of bullying and neglect. As a result of this, several hundred people are thought to have died linked to a variety of factors – from inadequately trained staff to a negative culture of care. This was attributed to low expectations and a lack of information sharing between various levels of health worker in the care of individual patients, a lack of professional commitment and poor communication between professionals, managers and the Trust Board. Although complaints were made repeatedly by patients' families, they were not taken seriously, nor taken forward with any urgency. There was a lack of leadership within the Trust and a lack of compassion was evident among the staff, including those providing hands-on care in support roles, as well as health professionals, managers and the Board – whose leadership was questioned.

Health support workers in the Trust had a critical role, but were often inadequately trained, supervised and managed by nurses and others within an unsupportive culture that fell short of acceptable standards. This was seen by the Inquiry as a significant contributory factor to the Trust's systemic failure. It was found that patients were not routinely assisted with toileting, frequently left in soiled clothes, and often not provided with water within reach. In short, their dignity and privacy were not respected. A number of recommendations were made in the interests of public and patient protection to reduce the risk of such poor levels of care. First and foremost, a set of well-publicised standards was required to ensure that all staff were caring, compassionate and considerate in their dealings with patients and their families. The maintenance of these standards was to be ensured through a rigorous system for regular monitoring and review, with clear lines of accountability for reports to named professional staff so the necessary action could be taken. It was held that those receiving treatment or care and their families must also be made aware of how to report any concerns. In addition, the Inquiry recommended that health support workers should be registered as qualified and have a uniform code of conduct. Frontline staff must be sufficiently well trained for their role and provided with opportunities for further educational development.

Despite the large numbers of health support workers, their vital contribution to the wellbeing of individual patients and their central importance to delivering health and social care services, effective policies to ensure suitability has been long delayed and there has been little research on the role they play. In a pioneering study undertaken some two decades ago, Saks and colleagues (2000) recommended an assessment of risk for this group and a route to a form of regulation. Their study was commissioned by the UK Departments of Health to review health support work. Their brief was to examine the roles, functions and responsibilities of support workers employed in health care settings, having due regard to the overlap of people who may also work in social care settings, and to make recommendations. In this study a support worker was defined as:

> A worker who provides face-to-face care or support of a personal or confidential nature to patients and/or service users in clinical or therapeutic settings, community facilities or domiciliary settings, but who does not hold qualifications accredited by a professional association and is not formally regulated by such a body (Saks et al 2000:21).

The study, described in the next section, focused on paid support workers, but at the request of government did not include the important army of unpaid volunteers, family members and other carers who had for long been known to provide much of the care in domiciliary settings (Finch and Groves 1983). The skills of health support workers were taken to include not only instrumental and technical skills, but also the normative, interactional and interpersonal skills of caring and empathy. Recent advertising material from the Royal College of Nursing and Midwifery (www.healthcareers.nhs. uk) aimed at recruiting health support workers has elaborated on the quality and skills required by support workers in nursing. In a somewhat confusing range of titles such as training nurse assistants and health care assistants, the range of tasks is described across various settings. For instance, in hospitals health support workers may deal with bodily maintenance tasks such as bathing, feeding and toileting, while in the community these roles may extend to a wider range of activities such as escorting users to community facilities.

The review by Saks and colleagues: risks, regulation and support workers

Data for the review by Saks and colleagues (2000) were gathered from a variety of sources, using mixed methods. A literature review was undertaken to gather the statistical data and other material on health support workers. A specially-designed structured questionnaire was sent out to the Chief Executives of all NHS trusts, health authorities, local authority social service departments and other mainstream bodies in the public, voluntary and private sector. Locality focus groups were also set up with participants from the public and private sector, including owners and managers of nursing and residential homes, users and carers, and health and social care support workers – in which risks and safeguards were among the key topics discussed. In addition, open regional workshops were held for stakeholder groups of support workers and professionals, employers and service providers, users and carers, and representative organisations covering the north, midlands and south of England, as well as Northern Ireland, Scotland and Wales. This complemented the in-depth individual interviews undertaken with several dozen influential stakeholders from professions, unions and other bodies at local, regional and national level. Finally, a website was set up for comment, to provide another data stream.

A main finding was that there were up to 1.5 million health support workers in the UK. This was a diverse group covering many hundreds of different occupational roles from health care assistants and nursing auxiliaries to occupational therapists and physiotherapy assistants. However, titles were not necessarily used consistently, nor were they indicative of the work undertaken. There was a large amount of part-time working and considerable movement between settings. In all, the number of health support workers was more than five times that of doctors and twice that of nurses in the UK. The invisible iceberg of health support workers thus formed the largest part of the health care workforce in both the public and private sector and in home, community and institutional settings.

From the evidence gathered, it was clear that there was no systematic regulatory framework for health support workers. This is not to say that there was no risk-oriented regulation at all, but this tended to occur at the level of local managers. For example, typically employers in organisational contexts would conduct pre-service checks to evaluate the suitability of health support workers. Normally regular supervision and/ or line management was carried out by qualified staff and development opportunities were provided by employers. National level legislation in areas such as employment, recruitment and safety at work covered health support workers as well as other employees. In addition, some voluntary registers existed for certain occupational groups. However, not all of these provisions were in place for every type of health support worker – especially for those working outside an agency framework and those who worked in people's own homes. A key question for the research was whether this was sufficiently robust to protect the people from harm and this was put to research participants in a survey.

In terms of risks to the public, most of the Chief Executives who responded to the survey felt that there were significant risks when support workers were employed. A quarter of respondents said the risks were considerable. Points of weakness in the existing system were seen to be the absence of codes of ethics to govern practice and the extremely limited use made of voluntary registers. These were not comprehensive and therefore not effective. In the focus groups three main types of risk were highlighted: how to identify unsuitable staff and so exclude them from the labour force; ambiguous role definitions that allowed the less well qualified to perform jobs beyond their competence; and the absence of standards for training and mechanisms to assess competence. Given these concerns, it was not surprising that a large majority of Chief Executives felt that there was a need for further regulation. In general, they supported more direct regulation overseen by a supervisory body and a mandatory register. The view was that this would bring greater consistency in the definition of roles and therefore improve standards and provide public protection from dangerous persons.

Feedback from the regional workshops also supported the case for a register of health support workers. It was felt that this would provide reassurance that employees were competent and reputable and would decrease the chances of unsuitable people moving from one post to another following a problem with an employer. To be sure, there were debates about entry requirements, registration mechanisms, information to be reported, and the costs involved. However, overall the view was that a transparent, user-friendly and efficient register, along with increased employer responsibilities underpinned by good practice standards, would be advantageous. Most employers commented that a register should be introduced within three years with support from the relevant trade unions. Both employers and health support worker staff commented that existing measures had emerged piecemeal, were inconsistent in the way they operated and did not give confidence in terms of public protection from risk.

On the basis of these findings, the review team recommended that there should be enhanced guidance for employees in health support roles; more active management and supervision of support workers by employers; and a clarification of employers' responsibilities. They also concluded that opportunities for training and career progression should be enhanced and that service users should be given more information on what to expect and an explanation of their rights. Finally, it was recommended that a register for health support workers should be introduced. Although the potential cost was acknowledged, it was suggested that a register could be phased in gradually. First, a simple register based on negative pre-service checks and regular monitoring of criminal records could be introduced, followed by a more comprehensive, mandatory, one-stop shop register for health support workers. A code of ethics could then be considered.

The review team was fully aware of the complexities of following this path. A minority of research participants were concerned about the administrative burden of further regulation and how employee checks might act as a deterrent to recruitment. The main obstacle was the cost of registration. While the cost of professional registration is borne by those wanting to register, it was unlikely that lower paid health support workers would be able to sustain a register through subscription. Government and employers would therefore have to contribute − even if a basic register was constructed. After lengthy internal debate, the government initially decided not to publish the review or introduce regulation despite the strong evidential base. Cost indeed seems to be the main reason for a lack of action. Permission to release the review was eventually obtained, the main findings and a summary from which are available in Saks and Allsop (2007).

The Cavendish review of risk, regulation and support workers

In the wake of the Francis report, the then Secretary of State for Health resurrected interest in risk and regulation related to health support workers by setting up an independent review of health and social care work led by Camilla Cavendish (2013). This review investigated the needs of the '1.3 million frontline staff who are not registered nurses but who now deliver the bulk of hands-on care in hospitals, care homes and the homes of individuals' (Cavendish 2013:5). Evidence was collected on the views of key players on topics such as recruitment, training, supervision, support and public confidence. The case for statutory registration was not investigated on the grounds that the Care Quality Commission, which monitors, inspects and regulates services in general practice, hospitals and care homes, provided sufficient protection to ensure that standards of quality and safety were being met. In our view, this takes an over-optimistic view of the capacity of those with responsibilities to monitor standards. The Care Quality Commission failed to spot problems at the Mid Staffordshire Trust and the poor standards of maternity care at Morecambe Bay. Visits from the Care Quality Commission are intermittent and the care provided by hospitals, care homes and domiciliary services in people's homes are often not integrated. Moreover, NHS contracts are notoriously difficult to terminate even if inadequate standards are identified.

The review by Cavendish (2013) placed an important emphasis on recruitment, training, education and career progression for health support workers. It recommended that a Certificate of Fundamental Care be introduced, with minimum, but quality-assured, training standards. It argued that support workers should complete the former before working unsupervised. Career progression should then be possible through a Higher Certificate of Fundamental Care with more advanced competences and further opportunities through various routes to NHS-funded courses and to nursing, social work and therapy degrees with the prospect of fast-tracking. The review stressed the importance of providing leadership and support, recommending that regulators, employers and commissioners should have common policies to relieve the pressure on first line managers and supervisors. It saw a role for the PSA in providing advice on employment matters, making referrals to other regulators and supporting the development of a generic code of conduct for both staff and employers. In addition, it suggested that the commissioning of support staff be based on the outcomes achieved, as opposed to data on activity alone. It also recommended that working conditions should be reviewed to consider payments for shift working and travel time.

Some years on, these recommendations have not been widely adopted (see, for instance, Ashurst 2015). However, Public Health England (2017) in a ten-year workforce strategy for health and social care follows through on some of the recommendations made by Cavendish. Nevertheless, after a long consultation phase and at the time of writing, a response from government has not been forthcoming. However, despite the lack of specific policies to regulate health support workers, there have been piecemeal attempts to increase the oversight of the health and social care sector in general. There is increased top-down regulation to enhance surveillance; a strengthening management oversight by both professional managers and administrators; and a stronger emphasis on training, education and career progression by national health and social care agencies, which has been enhanced by a growing focus on standards. We shall now turn to document aspects of this piecemeal approach before considering their reach in terms of ensuring quality of service, the safety of patients and their risk of harm.

Attempts to enhance the regulation of health support workers

In relation to top-down regulation, following the Bristol Inquiry and the case of Baby P, the Health Care Commission and the Commission for Social Care Inspection were established to oversee the health and social care sectors through setting standards and carrying out institutional visits. In 2009 the independent Care Quality Commission replaced these bodies and reports to government on care homes, hospitals, dental services, clinics, home care agencies, general practitioner services, mental health services and community-based health care services (Care Quality Commission 2018). However, as noted, the Commission has not been able to predict problems and prevent some serious breaches. Little is also known about the key risks of carers providing services in the home environment, not least where they are employed through private sector agencies. *Caveat emptor* applies as in any other open market transaction where contracting is undertaken by individual householders.

Nonetheless, in the health care sectors as a whole, professional bodies have decided to extend their remit to support the maintenance of quality standards among associates and accredited occupations. As Allsop and Jones (2018) relate, the PSA has prompted constituent professional Councils to address such issues as serial poor performance and criminal behaviour – and encourage clarity of process and the promotion of best practice. The PSA is an oversight and audit body with a comprehensive set of standards that follows the classic principles of proportionality, accountability, consistency, transparency and targeting promoted by the Better Regulation Task Force (2003). It claims to act proactively as well as reactively and uses a comparative method to compare the performance of Councils and promote learning of best practice (Professional Standards Authority 2015). Although its scale and powers have increased over time, central to its operation has been the notion of 'right-touch' regulation where the minimum regulatory force is used to achieve an outcome, taking risk into account. This may serve to protect the public and reduce risks associated with health professionals and those over whom it has oversight.

An increased focus on systems of management can also be seen as a positive process for ensuring quality and safety. This can take many forms. One type of systems management is the role that health professional regulatory Councils themselves play in developing the roles of associates and other interlinked support workers. Here the relevant Council plays a role in defining an area of work and accrediting qualifications and requirements for continuing professional development – as well as monitoring compliance for professionals on its register and associate professionals and, in some cases, professional assistants. These roles have been developed particularly by the medical, dental and nursing Councils. With regard to health support workers in the UK, employers in large organisations and small practices have an important management role in the selection, facilitation and oversight of the work of the occupational groups they employ. However, a challenge for management is that many support workers work across a number of settings and are employed part time. This may be by choice or due to a lack of alternatives.

Research to date suggests that the quality of management across organisations can vary and be a crucial factor in organisational performance (Kirkpatrick and Veronesi 2019). One example of variation in the degree to which new management systems are implemented effectively can be seen from research on the newly introduced system of periodic revalidation for doctors. A study by Archer and colleagues (2018) showed that revalidation had been accepted more positively in some NHS hospital trusts than others. Key factors influencing performance were well functioning IT systems that could bring data sets together to identify instances of recurrent complaints or incidents of poor practice, based on good working relationships between medical directors and managers. Management oversight has been found to be more difficult in smaller organisations such as hospices, primary care practices, private sector organisations and for doctors whose relationships to organisations has been more transient or distant, such as in locum services. Indeed, Waring and colleagues (2016) suggest that additional risks of poor practice are often due to human and localised environment factors. Much will depend on the skills of locally-based managers and supervisors and their commitment to a positive culture of quality improvement.

For other non-medical professions and occupations there has been little cohesive research on the effectiveness of either regulation or management on grass roots practice. Patients can 'voice' their concerns, pursue a complaint about poor practice or ultimately sue for negligence, but such actions are relatively rare and only taken after an adverse event has occurred. We now know more about the incidence of types of adverse event as possible indicators of risk, but data are complex and difficult to untangle. Moreover, they have weak predictive value (Lloyd-Bostock and Hutter 2008). In a recent exploratory study for the PSA, Searle and colleagues (2017) were asked to identify any pattern in the characteristics of professionals who had been the subject of a complaint called in and reviewed by the PSA as part of their oversight role of determinations by professional Councils in cases where a professional's continuing fitness-to-practice was being considered. The data consisted of several thousand determinations, covering doctors, nurses, social workers, paramedics and others. Some common factors were found in the background of those who had failed to provide an adequate service. Identification was made of the 'depleted perpetrator' as a professional who was struggling to deal with the pressures of life and the so-called, self-serving 'bad apple' who exploited the vulnerability of a client or patient in their own interest. There were also those practitioners whose work had been affected by a general fall in standards within their workplace. This classification suggests warning signs for service managers, although outside managed environments the onus for making judgements on the quality of service remains with patients and other clients.

Regulation can, therefore, only go so far in protecting users. It can be argued that health professionals, both doctors and others, may be less likely to provide an inadequate service as they are guided by clear ethical codes for their professional bodies and have a lengthy undergraduate education and common socialisation pattern as part of the process of professional registration (Saks 2015). Having said this, an effort was made in 2002 by the charitable not-for-profit sector to set national occupational standards for health and social care. Skills for Care (www. skillsforcare.org.uk) and Skills for Health (www.skillsforhealth.org.uk) both promote non-mandatory educational and training opportunities to enhance the quality of health care, even though their implementation has not been systematically monitored. For health support workers generally there is a greater reliance on management oversight to ensure an awareness of risks and guidance on ethical practice. The workforce consists of many diverse groups that operate in a range of settings and both managerial practice and opportunities for continuing education also vary. Overall, the care sector has tended to lag behind the health sector in the extent of regulatory oversight.

Conclusion: moving forward

While there have been advances in the regulation, management and education of professionals, associates and accredited occupations in the health and social care workforce, a report by Public Health England (2017) shows that most health support workers remain at the margin of these advances. This is despite the crucial role they play in meeting the needs of an ageing population with multiple chronic conditions and other vulnerable users (Saks 2008). We also do not know enough about this group to fully identify with confidence areas of risk that are a threat to patient safety. This raises the issue of what further regulation is required, what should be put in place to guide managers at the local level, and what education and opportunities for career progression should be provided in the client and public interest. At present regulatory confusion too often prevails in the division of labour in relation to support workers, who are themselves in a weak position in terms of market positioning.

In England in particular, one solution to mitigate the regulatory risks would be to establish a mandatory register for waged health support workers, as originally recommended by Saks and colleagues (2000). As they point out in their report, this could initially be a voluntary register that records and certifies the formal educational and training qualifications of support workers. While not being a fully-fledged professional register based on exclusionary closure, it could act as a one-stop repository for references, systematically guard against unspent criminal convictions, and prevent those struck off health professional registers from taking on health support worker roles. As such, it may have the added benefit of increasing the status and possibly the income of health support workers themselves. However, this raises the question of who pays the registration fee at a time when the income of this group is generally low (Barron and West 2013). Many health support workers are employed part time in precarious conditions (Cunningham et al 2016). Moreover, the experience of other countries in constructing such registers has not been wholly positive. In Ontario in Canada, for instance, the Ministry recently shut down its register, which had grown to include around one-third of the personal support workers in the province (Zlomislic 2016), even though currently consideration is being given to its resurrection.

This chapter has focused on policy developments in the UK with specific reference to England in the regulation of health support workers where there has been a distinct lack of progress in some areas, not least in contrast to Scotland where a Social Services Council register for support workers has recently been introduced and a code of conduct exists for health support workers. Nonetheless, the challenge of progressing health and social care services and the large workforce required is common in modern societies. We have shown that regulation for health and care professional and related occupational groups has moved forward, but further changes are required to enhance the quality of service standards and protect those in receipt of services from harm. Not all institutional changes have yet been sufficient or indeed effective. For instance, within the statutorily regulated professions, the scope of some regulatory Councils may be too large, such as in nursing, and in others it may be too small (Allsop and Jones 2018). Decisions made in the past about the location of particular occupations throw a long shadow forward. There is also uncertainty about the most appropriate organisational structure for some groups. For example, social work regained its independent status by separating from the HCPC towards the end of 2019 as a separate Council, Social Work England, with whatever implications this may bring.

Further investigation is undoubtedly required to fill gaps in our knowledge about the risks to users within each profession and occupation. We also need to know more about the views of the diverse range of such workers themselves on the hazards and stresses of their work world. In addition, there is an absence of knowledge about the views and experiences of those in receipt of health and social care services in an increasingly specialised division of labour where coordination has become a significant problem. If a register is not to be established for health support workers, ever greater weight should be given to the role of professionals and employers in providing support, supervision and management in a wider range of settings. This could be monitored by bodies like the Care Quality Commission and the PSA. There are lessons to be learned here for the limiting of risk not just for users and their carers on which this chapter has focused, but also – as other chapters have underlined – for the wellbeing of health support workers in face of the extremely stressful and difficult conditions under which many of them work.

References

Alaszewski, A. (2016) 'Risk, medicine and health', in Burgess, A., Alemanno, A. and Zinn, J.O. (eds) (2016) *The Routledge Handbook of Risk Studies*, Abingdon: Routledge.

Allsop, J. and Jones, K. (2018) 'Regulating the regulators: The rise of the Professional Standards Authority', in Chamberlain, J.M., Dent, M. and Saks, M. (eds) *Professional Health Regulation in the Public Interest: International Perspectives*, Bristol: Policy Press.

Allsop, J. and Saks, M. (eds) (2002) *Regulating the Health Professions*, London: Sage.

Archer, J., Bloor, K., Bojke, C., Boyd, A., Bryce, M., Ferguson, N., Gutacker, N., Hillier, C., Luscombe, K., Price, T., Regan de Bere, S., Tazzyman, A., Tredinnick-Rowe, J. and Walshe, K. (2018) *Evaluating the Development of Medical Revalidation in England and Its Impact on Organisational Performance and Medical Practice: Overview Report*, Manchester: University of Manchester/London: NIHR (PR-R-0114-11002).

Ashurst, A. (2015) 'How to … implement the Cavendish Review recommendations', *Nursing and Residential Care* 17(2): 115.

Askill, J. and Sharpe, M. (2014) *Angel of Death: Killer Nurse Beverly Allitt*, London: Michael O'Mara Books.

Barron, D.N. and West, E. (2013) 'The financial costs of caring in the British labour market: Is there a wage penalty for workers in caring occupations?', *British Journal of Industrial Relations* 51(1): 104–23.

Beck, U. (1992) *The Risk Society: Towards a New Modernity*, London: Sage.

Better Regulation Task Force (2003) *Principles of Good Regulation*, London: Better Regulation Task Force.

Burgess, A. (2016) 'Introduction', in Burgess, A., Alemanno, A. and Zinn, J.O. (eds) (2016) *The Routledge Handbook of Risk Studies*, Abingdon: Routledge.

Care Quality Commission (2018) *Annual Report and Accounts 2017/18*, London: Care Quality Commission.

Cavendish, C. (2013) *An Independent Review into Healthcare Assistants and Support Workers in the NHS and Social Care Settings*, https://assets.publishing.service.gov.uk/government/uploads/system/uploads/attachment_data/file/236212/Cavendish_Review.pdf

Chamberlain, J.M. (2015) *Medical Regulation, Fitness to Practise and Revalidation*, Bristol: Policy Press.

Cunningham, I., Baines, D., Shields, J. and Lewchuk, W. (2016) 'Austerity policies, "precarity" and the nonprofit workforce: A comparative study of UK and Canada', *Journal of Industrial Relations* 58(4): 455–72.

Department of Health (2000) *A Health Service of All the Talents: Developing the NHS Workforce*, London: The Stationery Office.

Department of Health (2006a) *Good Doctors, Safer Patients. Proposals to Strengthen the System to Assure and Improve the Performance of Doctors and to Protect the Safety of Patients: A Report by the Chief Medical Officer*, London: The Stationery Office.

Department of Health (2006b) *The Regulation of the Non-medical Healthcare Professions: A Review by the Department of Health*, London: The Stationery Office.

Department of Health (2007) *Trust Assurance and Safety: The Regulation of Health Professionals in the 21st Century*, London: The Stationery Office.

Esland, G. (1980) 'Diagnosis and therapy', in Esland, G. and Salaman, G. (eds) *The Politics of Work and Occupations*, Milton Keynes: Open University Press.

Finch, J. and Groves, D. (eds) (1983) *Labour of Love: Women, Work and Caring*, London: Routledge and Kegan Paul.

Francis, R. (2013) *Report of the Mid Staffordshire NHS Foundation Trust Public Inquiry*, London: The Stationery Office, www.gov.uk/government/publications/report-of-the-mid-staffordshire-nhs-foundation-trust-public-inquiry

General Medical Council (2018) *Annual Report 2017*, London: GMC.

General Social Care Council (2004) *Corporate Plan 2004–05 to 2006–07*, London: GSCC.

Goode, W.J. (1960) 'Encroachment, charlatanism and the emerging profession: Psychology, sociology and medicine', *American Sociological Review* 25: 902–14.

Ham, C. (2009) *Health Policy in Britain*, Basingstoke: Palgrave Macmillan.

Johnson, T. (1995) 'Governmentality and the institutionalization of expertise', in Johnson, T., Larkin, G. and Saks, M. (eds) *Health Professions and the State in Europe*, London: Routledge.

Jones, R. (2014) *Baby P: Setting the Record Straight*, Bristol: Policy Press.

Kirkpatrick, I. and Veronesi, G. (2019) 'Researching health care management using secondary data', in Saks, M. and Allsop, J. (eds) *Researching Health: Qualitative, Quantitative and Mixed Methods*, 3rd edition, London: Sage.

Kirkup, B. (2015) *The Report of the Morecambe Bay Investigation*, London: The Stationery Office.

Klein, R. (2013) *The New Politics of the NHS: From Creation to Reinvention*, 7th edition, London: Radcliffe Publishing.

Lloyd-Bostock, S. and Hutter, B.H. (2008) 'Reforming regulation in the medical profession: The risks of risk-based approaches', *Health, Risk and Society* 10(1): 69–83.

McKee, M., Dubois, C.-A. and Sibbald, B. (2006) 'Changing professional boundaries', in Dubois, C.-A., McKee, M. and Nolte, E. (eds) *Human Resources for Health in Europe*, Maidenhead: Open University Press.

Professional Standards Authority (2015) *Annual Report 2014/2015*, London: PSA.

Public Health England (2017) *Facing the Facts, Shaping the Future: A Draft Health and Care Workforce Strategy for England to 2027*, London: Health Education England.

Roche, W. (2018) 'Medical regulation for the public interest in the United Kingdom', in Chamberlain, J.M., Dent, M. and Saks, M. (eds) *Professional Health Regulation in the Public Interest: International Perspectives*, Bristol: Policy Press.

Saks, M. (2008) 'Policy dynamics: Marginal groups in the healthcare division of labour in the UK', in Kuhlmann, E. and Saks, M. (eds) *Rethinking Professional Governance: International Directions in Healthcare*, Bristol: Policy Press.

Saks, M. (2010) 'Analyzing the professions: The case for a neo-Weberian approach', *Comparative Sociology* 9(6): 887–915.

Saks, M. (2015) *The Professions, State and the Market: Medicine in Britain, the United States and Russia*, Abingdon: Routledge.

Saks, M. (2016a) 'The regulation of the English health professions: Zoos, circuses or safari parks?', in Liljegren, A. and Saks, M. (eds) *Professions and Metaphors: Understanding Professions in Society*, Abingdon: Routledge.

Saks, M. (2016b) 'Review of theories of professions, organizations and society: Neo-Weberianism, neo-institutionalism and eclecticism', *Journal of Professions and Organization* 3(2): 170–87.

Saks, M. and Allsop, J. (2007) 'Social policy, professional regulation and health support work in the United Kingdom', *Social Policy and Society* 6(2): 165–77.

Saks, M., Allsop, J., Chevannes, M., Clark, M., Fagan, R., Genders, N., Johnson, M., Kent, J., Payne, C., Price, D., Szczepura, A. and Unell, J. (2000) *Review of Health Support Workers. Report to the UK Departments of Health*, Leicester: UK Departments of Health/De Montfort University.

Searle, R.H., Rice, C., McConnell, A.A. and Dawson, J.F. (2017) *Bad Apples? Bad Barrels? Or Bad Cellars? Antecedents and Processes of Professional Misconduct in UK Health and Social Care: Insights into Sexual Misconduct and Dishonesty*, Coventry: Coventry University.

Smith, J. (2004) *The Shipman Inquiry: Fifth Report: Safeguarding Patients: Lessons from the Past – Proposals for the Future*, London: The Stationery Office.

Walshe, K., Boyd, A., Bryce, M., Luscombe, K., Tazzyman, A., Tredinnick-Rowe, J. and Archer, J. (2016) 'Implementing medical revalidation in the United Kingdom: Findings about organisational changes and impacts from a survey of Responsible Officers', *Journal of the Royal Society of Medicine* 110(1).

Waring, J., Allen, D., Braithwaite, J. and Sandall, J. (2016) 'Healthcare quality and safety: A review of policy, practice and research', *Sociology of Health and Illness* 38(2): 198–215.

Zlomislic, D. (2016) 'Ontario closes personal support worker register', *Toronto Star* 27 January.

Note: The authors would like to give their thanks to Marc Seale, Chief Executive of the Health and Care Professions Council in the UK, for reading and commenting on an earlier draft of this chapter. The contents of this chapter, however, remain the sole responsibility of the authors.

SIX

The interface of health support workers with the allied health professions

Susan Nancarrow

Introduction

This chapter describes the way the health support workforce interfaces with allied health professions, first through an international perspective, and then with greater focus on the UK and Australian contexts. Allied health practitioners have been working with support workers since at least the mid-20th century (Salvatori 2001), with evidence of formal training for occupational therapy assistants in the United States as early as the 1950s – while several professions saw a proliferation of assistants during the early 1970s in Canada and the UK (Robinson et al 1994; Webb et al 2004). Since then, despite varying levels of opposition from professional bodies and inconsistent access to training and professional support, support workers are now a key component of many health and social services contributing to the care provided by a wide range of allied health disciplines (Farndon and Nancarrow 2003; Saks and Allsop 2007; Salvatori 2001). As a result, support workers are a growing and increasingly diverse group of practitioners supporting the delivery of various allied health services.

Allied health support workers have been introduced primarily as a way to increase allied health capacity to meet the needs of an expanding and ageing population and to account for a shortfall in professionally qualified practitioners (Salvatori 2001). They have also been seen as an economically effective way to deliver safe and skilled care, while enabling the professional workforce to upskill to provide more specialist services (Foster 2006). The support worker role is therefore seen as a way to free up the time for allied health professionals to carry out more complex tasks by maintaining or increasing the capacity of care previously delivered by professionally qualified practitioners (Pullenayegum et al 2005; Stanmore et al 2005). Consequently, the expansion of support workers has been a focus of recent health workforce reform in the UK and various Australian states with policies targeting growth in numbers, expansion of roles and the introduction of new types of roles (Saks and Allsop 2007; Wanless 2002).

One challenge of understanding the support workforce associated with allied health is the lack of central coordination. Consequently numerous roles, models and worker titles have emerged (Bach et al 2008; Buchan and Dal Poz 2002; Lizarondo et al 2010; Saks and Allsop 2007). There is also evidence that support worker roles are highly context specific (Nancarrow 2004). Given the same title or grade, an assistant in one setting may carry out different roles and duties to those in a different setting. Additionally, the heterogeneity of the allied health workforce means that support work is necessarily fragmented and it is difficult to make generalisations. To date, the support worker role has not been subject to statutory regulation or training in Australia or the UK; instead their clinical governance tends to fall under particular jurisdictional arrangements. The lack of regulation and formalisation of qualifications means that there is no clearly defined scope of practice, thus limiting more overarching statements regarding the types of support work performed and the transferability of support worker roles.

The influence of context on roles is important. The largely localised development of support workers means their roles are defined by the tasks allocated by the allied health staff with whom they work. Delegation to support workers, however, is a complex and multifaceted process which further influences the variety of such roles depending on factors like a qualified professional assessment or judgement about the experience and competence of the support worker (Ellis and Connell 2001; Hancock et al 2005; Hek et al 2004; Mackey and Nancarrow 2005; Ormandy et al 2004; Spilsbury and Meyer 2005; Stanmore and Waterman 2007). Additionally, the range of settings in which support workers deliver care has an important impact on their roles. Shifting care away from the organisational hierarchy of the hospital into the community or patients' own homes provides a radical departure from the traditional institutionally-bound divisions of labour, control of technology and determination of roles (Turner 1995; Zagrodney and Saks 2017).

The chapter will first describe the allied health workforce, then explore the evolution of the support workforce associated with the allied health professions, including the drivers for the introduction of a support workforce, the contexts in which support workforce are employed and the negotiation of their boundaries, and the challenges and opportunities for both allied health professions and the support workforce. Specifically, this chapter argues that the allied health support workforce has evolved through two specific models, resulting in different types of workers. The first is the profession-led model, which supports the neo-Weberian idea of the professional project outlined by Larson (1977), in which the allied health professions developed support roles as a way to expand and maintain their market monopoly and professional autonomy in niche areas. The second is the managerial model, which moves away from the primacy of the profession and instead privileges 'patient-centred' goals of increasing role flexibility by recognising and rewarding individuals' skills and competencies rather than professional titles – and works across traditional professional and organisational boundaries.

What is allied health?

To explore the interrelationship between allied health and their associated support workforce first requires an explanation of the complex federation of professions that comprise allied health. Collectively, allied health professionals provide a broad range of services in acute care, aged care, rehabilitation, diagnosis, health promotion, early intervention, oral health and mental health. They tend to be autonomous practitioners who can work alone or in multidisciplinary teams with an emphasis on preventative as well as diagnostic and therapeutic services. Despite several attempts to define allied health professions through specific inclusion and exclusion criteria, as well as different philosophical approaches and clinical techniques (Olson 2012; Turnbull et al 2009), there is no single accepted taxonomy or definition of allied health professionals. The term allied health now is widely used in Anglo-American countries to encompass a range of health professions that are not nursing or medicine.

NHS England recognises 14 allied health profession groups, namely art therapists, drama therapists, music therapists, chiropodists/podiatrists, dietitians, occupational therapists, operating department practitioners, orthoptists, osteopaths, paramedics, physiotherapists, prosthetists and orthotists, radiographers, and speech and language therapists. There is no nationally accepted definition of allied health within Australia. However, allied health generally excludes paramedics and operating department practitioners, but may include audiology, psychology, social work, pharmacy, radiation therapists, medical laboratory scientists, as well as osteopaths and chiropractors despite their early explicit exclusion (Willis 1983). Definitions in the United States, Canada and New Zealand are similarly diverse (Astley 2000; Lecca et al 2003). The reliability of information available on allied health is further inhibited by a lack of systematic definitions and approaches to data collection and a literature that is lacking in historic analysis and detail (Nancarrow et al 2017; Olson 2012; Ottosson 2016; Willis 1983).

The attributes of the allied health professions that are important in terms of their relationship to support workers include the determination of allied health roles under the patronage of the medical profession; their adoption of a niche area of expertise (rather than the broader repertoire of nursing and medicine); their regulation, either by the state or by a governing professional body; and their typical involvement in state service provision and management (Larkin 2002), although they may also practise autonomously under a fee-for-service model in a cluster of professions that are strongly female dominated (Nancarrow et al 2017; Ottosson 2016). As such, allied health professions occupy an interesting space within the medical division of labour. While some of these professions existed prior to the establishment of the General Medical Council in 1858, the subsequent evolution of the allied health professions has involved careful negotiation about professional scopes of practice under the watchful patronage of the medical profession (Larkin 1983; Willis 1983). In return for medical patronage, allied health roles were clearly defined by the medical profession, often through legislation or regulation. As a result, the allied health professions were subject to role limitation and subordinated to medical control in neo-Weberian terms as medicine sought to exercise its authority and shape the division of labour (Turner 1985, 1995).

Unlike medicine and nursing with strong brand recognition, large professional size, internal hierarchies, recognised specialisms and a strong political voice, the allied health professions are a federation of independent disciplines, each of varying size, focusing on niche areas of practice (Larkin 1995). The scale and internal professional hierarchies of nursing and medicine are also importantly distinct from those of the allied health professions. Internal professional hierarchies provide a way for medicine and nursing to incorporate new skills into their professional repertoire through a division of labour, effectively increasing the scope of their professional practice. In contrast, allied health professions have few formally recognised specialisms within their divisions of labour. Therefore, professional advancement is largely based on managerial structures (McClimens et al 2010). The implications of this are twofold. First, the nature of the clinical tasks that can be delegated by allied health professionals falls within a narrow scope of practice derivative from the niche offering of specific allied health professions. For example, physiotherapy assistants tend to be delegated repetitive, hands-on technical tasks that form the core of the physiotherapists' repertoire alongside a range of administrative tasks (Ellis and Connell 2001). Second, allied health professions lack the internal professional career hierarchies enabling them to advance professionally within an internal division of labour as they cast off unwanted tasks to lower grade staff in their own division of labour, losing the advantages of delegation in the large professional hierarchies of medicine and nursing.

This has important implications for the development of the allied health support workforce. While the medical and nursing professions have been able to achieve upward and outward expansion of their professional repertoires through specialisation and subordination of the workforce in their division of labour, the contract between the medical profession and the allied health professions has effectively limited any vertical mobility that creates direct competition with the medical profession (Larkin 1983). Thus, as allied health professions have expanded their repertoires through access to modalities such as prescribing, it has had little effect on their professional structures. Consequently, like the adoption of technical roles in nursing, the employment of a support workforce may erode core allied health work without the concomitant expansion of their own professional repertoire (Davies 1995). Moreover, the heterogeneity of the allied health professions means associated support workers, who are predominantly unregulated and locally grown, have even more diverse and complex positions. Rather than attempt to address issues specific to every allied health discipline, this chapter draws on published accounts of support worker roles associated with the allied health disciplines and brings out issues and themes that are common across jurisdictions and professions.

The development of the support workforce for the allied health professions

While the allied health support workforce has existed since the latter half of the 20th century (Ellis and Connell 2001; Salvatori 2001; Webb et al 2004), the focus on it has increased as health services adopt an increasingly managerial agenda and recognise opportunities for efficiencies while reorienting care around more patient-centred principles. As noted, the allied health support workforce has evolved through two distinct models. The first is the profession-driven model, the earliest model of the development of allied health support workers with the delegation of roles to auxiliaries under the direction of allied health professionals. The second is the managerial model, which has become increasingly dominant during the late 20th and early 21st century, as large-scale workforce reform brought about centralised support and development for support worker roles across a range of settings and jurisdictions – and the emergence of a suite of tools re-engineered the workforce around patient needs and risk, rather than professional preferences.

The two processes are not entirely independent, as the managerial agenda has, in some cases, supported professional goals of growth for the allied health professions, or indeed driven the introduction of profession specific support workers, as was the case with podiatry assistants (Webb et al 2004). However, increasingly the managerial agenda has taken the responsibility for role renegotiation out of the hands of the professions and placed it under the development of bureaucracies (Dent et al 2004). Furthermore, both approaches involve the codification and devolution of tasks from qualified allied health practitioners to support workers, even if each approach has a different driver, and the results are different. Under the profession–driven model the drivers largely involve increasing the capacity of the profession in the division of labour of a single profession, primarily through the delegation of unwanted tasks under the direct supervision of an allied health professional. This provides increased opportunities for professionals to focus on more highly skilled, generally less technical, tasks and to increase the volume of patients. In comparison, managerial drivers are bureaucratically inspired and more patient focused, with a less clear division of labour and ownership of tasks and a greater likelihood of involving the devolution of tasks from specific professions in a generic model of working. These approaches are now explored more fully.

The profession-driven model of allied health support worker development

The profession-driven model of support worker development was documented as early as the 1950s in occupational therapy in Canada (Salvatori 2001) and, later, in physiotherapy and podiatry in the NHS in the UK (Webb et al 2004). The early introduction of discipline specific allied health support workers was primarily promoted to increase the capacity of already stretched allied health professions and to allow existing practitioners to focus on more highly skilled areas of practice, while delegating unwanted or more routine tasks (Le Cornu et al 2010). However, there was also early recognition that the use of therapy aides was a professionalisation strategy. One example is the podiatry assistant role, first formally introduced in response to podiatry workforce shortages in England by the NHS in 1977, initially as foot hygienists under the supervision of podiatrists (Webb et al 2004). The role was also proposed to stop podiatrists performing tasks which did not require their level of expertise. It initially met with resistance from the profession because of concerns about competition from podiatrists working in the private sector, patients being put at risk, and the protection of the professional status of podiatrists.

The history of allied health support workers in Australia is poorly documented, but they were more recently introduced than in the UK or North America. This was likely due to the high proportion of allied health professions in private practice, and resistance to competition by their professional bodies. Prior to the introduction of podiatry assistants, a shortage of podiatry services in Australia resulted in the delegation of basic foot care services to enrolled nurses managed in the nursing division of labour (Moran et al 2012). This meant that podiatrists lost control over a component of their core business to the larger group of nurses, and their patients were managed under the nursing, not podiatry, team. This created a disjointed service pathway and clinical governance concerns about foot care services – as well as unhappiness among some enrolled nurses about being delegated the low status, discarded foot care role. A parallel analysis of the employment of foot care assistants in the UK (Farndon and Nancarrow 2003) found some podiatry services did not employ foot care assistants because of a focus on 'high risk' patients, at the expense of 'low risk' podiatry work, including basic foot care and nail maintenance – on which delegation to foot care assistants by other services was centred. The use of foot care assistants here was seen to increase the opportunities for podiatrists to specialise. However, none of the 'specialisations' identified were formally recognised and most were extensions of the existing scope of practice of podiatrists. Instead, the use of foot care assistants enabled podiatrists in larger departments to concentrate on niche areas of interest, while delegating, or ignoring, the low status, low risk tasks.

Both of these examples demonstrate how podiatrists lost professional control of a component of their work during a time of workforce shortages. In Australia the service was delivered outside the supervision of podiatrists as they surrendered their division of labour to nurses – illustrating the importance of employing auxiliaries within the scope of practice of the allied health practitioners. The podiatrists in this example were able to regain control over their core business through the re-allocation of roles to newly developed support workers because nurses and podiatrists were employed within the same community organisation. However, had the enrolled nurses been employed separately, it is possible that the roles would not have been returned.

Interestingly, the introduction of the podiatry assistant did not impact the workload of podiatrists because it only resulted in the transfer of foot care work previously performed by enrolled nurses. In the UK low risk foot care was deemed by podiatrists to be of sufficiently low priority and status to completely disregard this work. The services that employed podiatry assistants maintained such foot care within their division of labour. However, other services effectively dropped this low risk, low status work from their repertoire to focus on higher risk and status 'virtuoso' roles such as diabetes management and biomechanics (Hugman 1991). This was despite the concerns from private podiatrists that unregulated practitioners would step in and take over basic foot care.

As with podiatry assistants in the UK, their establishment in Australia met with mixed responses from the profession. The issues facing podiatry assistants are reminiscent of the tensions created by the early introduction of most allied health support worker roles. These focused on resisting threats to the monopolies of the allied professions through boundary maintenance and the creation of status hierarchies through the development of subordinate grades subject to the control of professionals (Webb et al 2004). Opponents to support workers in many allied health professions expressed concerns that the introduction of support workers was merely a way to provide allied health care at a lower cost, leading to deprofessionalisation (Braverman 1974; Le Cornu et al 2010). The dietetic support worker, recently introduced by the British Dietetics Association to reduce the increasing incidence of malnutrition among hospital in-patients, provides a different example. This role was in fact led by the profession, drawing on successful models of support worker implementation from the United States. It reflected the changing socio-political landscape in following the introduction of the evidence-based medicine movement and in responding to perceived service needs, including efficiency and patient-centred values supported by the managerial agenda (Le Cornu et al 2010). The role of dietetic support worker therefore met with little professional resistance, as it fell within tightly constrained boundaries under the supervisory control of the dietetics profession.

This analysis of the profession-driven model of allied health support worker development fits readily with neo-Weberianism, in which professions attempt to control their role and task boundaries to their own advantage in terms of status, income and power (Allsop and Saks 2002; Larkin 1988; Macdonald 1995). As the case of podiatrists in the UK and Australia highlights, allied health professions can surrender as well as gain market position if they lose control over their core work at a time of a shortage of supply. What is less clear is the ability of the profession to recoup or extend their skills or tasks during times of workforce abundance (Nancarrow and Borthwick 2005). Professions therefore need to be looking to expand their repertoire upwards at the same time as delegating to support workers. Unlike the medical profession, which has relied on the subordination of auxiliary professions to enable them to define the scope of new, specialised medical roles (Johnson 2016), the allied health professions have largely used the opportunity of having subordinate staff to adopt a narrower focus of work falling within their existing scope of practice. In this vein, the recent expansion of the scope of allied health professionals into prescribing – as a previous territory of medicine and nursing – has not significantly increased their status or stature as specialists.

The employment setting plays an important role in the structure of the work of allied health professionals, and their subsequent division of labour in the profession-driven model. Most of the documented examples of the introduction of allied health support workers have been implemented within bureaucracies, not in fee-for-service private practices, although there is evidence of private practitioners employing support workers. For instance, in an Australian study by the Victorian Department of Health and Human Services (2016) some 60 per cent of physiotherapists reported working with allied health assistants and of these, 10 per cent of these were in the private sector. Practitioners working within bureaucracies have different drivers to those working in fee-based private practice as they have a pecuniary interest in ensuring that they optimise their income. This involves reducing competition and increasing throughput. Conversely, practitioners working in a bureaucracy, such as a hospital or community setting, may be driven stronger by service goals and targets, even though these may be increasingly likely to involve patient throughput and productivity and efficiency drivers.

The managerial model of allied health support worker development

The managerialist agenda, or the New Public Management, emerged from New Right market policies designed to increase the efficient and effective use of resources, while reducing professional power and clinical freedom by empowering non-medical managers of services across professional boundaries (Dent et al 2004; Ham 1994; Salter 2001; Strong and Robinson 1990). The effects of the managerialist agenda on the professions have been widely debated

(Noordegraaf 2007), although in health care the exploration tends to focus on larger professions such as medicine and nursing (see, for example, Carvalho 2014), with limited attention paid to allied health professions.

The debates around the effects of managerialism revisit the definitions of a profession (Noordegraaf 2007) or attempt to redefine the meaning of profession in a changing environment (Evetts 2006). The subordinate professional emergence of the allied health professions in the medical division of labour is one of their defining features, distinguishing them from medical colleagues (Larkin 1983). Again the exploration of deprofessionalisation has largely centred on the medical profession (Saks 2015), where there is some evidence that managerialism has diminished autonomy and eroded rewards. However, no health care professions have as willingly fragmented their core business to others to the extent undertaken by the allied health professions, which have actively developed tools to aid the disaggregation and re-engineering of their roles to meet managerial objectives (Smith and Duffy 2010). Here the managerial values of individual responsibility and fiscal probity have driven policies which sought to empower patients and constrain public expenditure (Malin et al 2002; Pollock 2004). Increasing emphasis on user involvement and consumer choice shifted the focus of health care provision towards the principles of self-management, health education and early intervention away from hospital treatment (Alaszewski 1995; Allsop 1995).

Under New Labour, the NHS Modernisation Agenda and NHS Plan in the UK (Department of Health 2000) were key policy instruments of the managerial agenda, supported by National Service Frameworks. This approach – which has been variously built on by subsequent political regimes such as the Coalition and the Conservative government (see, for example, Klein 2013) – were the drivers for managerial values based on user-centred care and patient choice. These have underpinned a health-focused service that engages people in living healthier lives, with quality targets to improve timely access to care, efficiency and sustainability through new financing mechanisms such as payment by results; new commissioning models that include joint ventures with the independent sector; care closer to home; and partnership working through legislation enabling local authorities and health authorities to share resources. This is part of the shifting health policy landscape which Saks (2016b) metaphorically describes as having changed from zoos with self-regulatory health professions to circuses where government acts like a ringmaster in regulating the professions and now safari parks characterised by efforts to bring health and social care together.

Alongside targets to increase existing workforce capacity through expanded training places, recruitment and retention strategies, a number of new roles were introduced in the UK that could respond quickly to changing workforce needs, while addressing the shifting values of the managerial agenda. These included the explicit, centralised development of roles such as assistant practitioners, consultant therapists and support workers in intermediate care. The NHS Modernisation Agency (2004) introduced the Changing Workforce Programme which pioneered and implemented role redesign in line with new values. This included vertically shifting tasks up or down a traditional unidisciplinary ladder; expanding the breadth of existing roles; increasing the depth of existing roles; and developing new jobs by combining existing tasks in new ways. The ageing population was a specific target for service modernisation, resulting in the rapid emergence of new models of care such as intermediate care designed to support older people through their illness trajectory by integrating services around patient needs and introducing services to support rehabilitation and the management of long-term conditions. Each of these services was specifically relevant to the remit of allied health, and consequently associated support worker staff operating under a managerial approach.

A range of role redesign projects were undertaken in England using a fast-track approach. These included the development of assistants to allied health professionals such as generic rehabilitation assistants, who could provide a seven-day service to support allied health professionals in rehabilitation and intermediate care at home. An example of the large-scale engineering of support workers to meet the needs of older people in intermediate care services was the Accelerated Development Programme in Intermediate Care (Nancarrow et al 2005). This programme involved the rapid and systematic implementation of new support roles across 50 intermediate care services in England, including rehabilitation assistants, home care support workers and early discharge workers. It aimed to increase the capacity of older peoples' services; reduce avoidable admissions to acute hospitals for older people; and minimise premature or avoidable dependence on long-term care in institutional settings. These support roles were designed to sit across a range of professional repertoires to reduce the number of different staff seen by the same service user, while leading to more effective use of a clinician's time. At the same time, nationally recognised qualifications for support workers, such as foundation degrees and National Vocational Qualifications, were introduced.

The proportion of support staff to professionally qualified staff varied widely between services, but across the services involved there were, on average, two support workers employed for every professionally qualified practitioner. Different agencies could host the intermediate care services, including primary health care, social services and acute services, as well as multiple agency partnerships – typically between primary care and social services. The multi-agency focus of the services meant support workers were employed in diverse host organisations. This was reflected in team leadership, which included nurses, allied health professionals, social workers, support workers and home care workers. Kessler and Bach (2007) highlighted the important role of support workers as boundary spanners, brokering transitions across disciplines, agencies, settings and class structures within this managerialist approach. In intermediate care, support workers were developed outside the scope of practice or specific disciplines, and were engineered to sit across multiple traditional roles and more closely align with the patient, while brokering relationships with members of the multidisciplinary team. Such boundary spanning roles are now seen as a core component of health service integration (Gilburt 2016).

Importantly, most of the intermediate care services were delivered in the patient's own home, providing a practical imperative for minimising the number of different practitioners involved in the care of an individual patient. The home-based setting of intermediate care support workers was an important facilitator of the support worker role (Nancarrow 2004). The practicality of delivering care in the patient's own home meant that visiting practitioners were often 'solo practitioners' in that context, so that support workers could be called on to undertake tasks that would normally fall beyond the scope of a single practitioner. Tasks were therefore delegated to support workers from a range of professions, including physiotherapists, dietitians and occupational therapists. Similarly, the goals of patients at home tended to reflect their interaction with, and ability to function within, their environment, rather than more technical goals defined by the therapist.

In the profession-driven approach, the setting of care is an important determinant of worker roles, with a focus on the hospital reinforcing the hierarchies and dominance of the medical profession (Turner 1995). The internal governance of hospitals in the managerial approach is underlined by the concept of a hospital as a rational bureaucracy in which specialised duties are formally defined and performed in a stable and systematic manner, overseen by management officials. The shift of care into the home creates an even more ideal environment in which the managerial agenda can be implemented, with the patient at the centre and the home as the workplace (England and Dyck 2011). Symbolic indicators of a shift in power towards the patient include keeping patient notes at the home; the importance of the support worker in determining the health care needs of the patient, in contrast to the doctor or nurse at the hospital bedside; and the lack of hospital technology in the home as a therapeutic environment. Freidson (1970) has observed that clinicians working in isolation from colleagues were more likely to develop patient-dependent, as opposed to colleague-dependent, practice.

The type of care also influences the role of support workers. More acute models of care for patients with high level needs are shorter term and demand more regular input from more highly skilled staff. In this context, support workers have less input and tend to receive more tightly specified tasks. In contrast, longer-term Hospital at Home services provide opportunities for more task delegation to support workers, as well as more joint visits by therapists (England and Dyck 2011). In this case, the level of patient dependency necessitates a more formal care hierarchy and division of roles. A further consideration of patient centredness is the social status of the health worker relative to the patient. The status of professions has long been linked with that of their associates and patients or clients. Indeed, the dominance of the medical profession was initially enhanced by the elevated position of their patients. Similarly, the early development of physiotherapy received royal patronage and was linked to well-to-do clients, which substantially increased the standing of the profession (Larkin 1983). However, with support workers, the converse may be true. In Staffordshire in the UK, for example, occupational therapy assistant practitioner roles were developed to provide work for local factory hands following the closure of the potteries (Nancarrow and Mackey 2005). Their class background and a lack of university education, though, meant that assistant practitioners 'spoke a different language' to qualified occupational therapists:

However, within the occupational therapy service, managers recognised that class and language barriers between qualified and unqualified staff could enhance the relationships between assistant practitioners and users as the support workers were representatives of the communities they served, rather than those of professions. The role of language in asserting professional power and occupational hierarchies is well documented (Saks 2016a). However, the managerial agenda forcibly undermined class agendas by shifting health care delivery from powerful elites to auxiliaries and lay people and even the lay workforce. The health care division of labour is also heavily influenced within the managerial model by different perspectives on types of illness and associated health care activities. Within the medical profession, the status of different specialities varies according to activity (Shortell 1974). Lower skilled or esteemed tasks are more likely to be delegated to others. The complexity of work also influences its status (Abbott 1981), where 'routine', or less complex, work is more likely to be managed by lower status professions, in contrast to more complex, 'less routine', tasks which are more likely to be referred to a specialist practitioner (Friedson 1970). Abbott (1981) takes the concept of intraprofessional status further, proposing that it is a function of 'professional purity', in which the highest status professionals deal with the most processed issues and problems, which have had human complexity removed by others. Conversely, lowest status work involves the greatest human complexity as illustrated by support workers in the home care setting. The case of support workers in intermediate care is the ultimate expression of the managerial rather than profession-driven approach.

Challenges faced by the allied health support workforce

The previous section has focused on the UK, in part because in Australia the centralised introduction and implementation of allied health support worker roles has largely been led at the level of state health departments, reflecting the devolved Australian funding model – where medical services are predominantly funded by the federal government and allied health and community services by the state. Each state has developed and introduced its own guidelines on the development of support workers. However, some managerial centralisation of role development is still evident. The interdisciplinary consensus approach is illustrated by the introduction of support workers by Queensland Health which undertook a Delphi study of key stakeholders to determine which roles could be delegated (Stute et al 2013). While support worker roles are well established in the UK, though, the allied health support workforce is still developing, primarily due to the changing contexts in which it operates. Several issues facing this workforce are common across roles and jurisdictions. Some of the most significant are set out in the following itinerary.

Quality and inconsistency of training

Training for allied health support workers is still inconsistent and confusing, particularly in Australia with its less centralised approach to allied health support workers. While there are large variations, the models of support worker training tend to involve generic vocational training, supported by in-house, context specific training (Nancarrow and Mackey 2005). Several studies of support workers have reported the challenges posed by support workers undertaking non-standardised qualifications. The challenges stem from a lack of clear role identity, visibility, transferability of roles and clarity of title. A traineeship model which interspersed formal vocational qualification and on-the-job training that was led by speech language pathologists resulted in a clearer relationship with support workers and a clearer understanding of the activities that could be performed (Nancarrow et al 2015).

Lack of career progression opportunities

Opportunities for career progression are generally limited for allied health support workers for two reasons. As McClimens and colleagues (2010) document, the first is the lack of profession-based hierarchies as in most allied health professions. The second challenge is a lack of appropriate career pathways to facilitate the transition from a support role to a professionally qualified role. Despite numerous attempts to introduce career pathways for allied health support workers to become qualified allied health practitioners, there are few exemplars of effective transition. The challenge seems to be that the qualifications required to become an allied health support worker are inconsistent with the entry level qualifications to an undergraduate allied health training programme. However, the so-called 'step-on, step-off' pathways develop practitioners who are overqualified to work as a support worker, but underqualified to work as an allied health practitioner.

Inefficient delegation

One of the most common challenges reported by support workers is the inconsistency and inefficiency of delegation by allied health practitioners. This tends to arise due to confusion around who is accountable for outcomes, and concern about risks that may arise if an allied health practitioner delegates activities to support workers. As Mackey and Nancarrow (2005) indicate, the lack of role clarity and definition means that allied health staff do not have a consistent understanding of the capabilities of the support worker until they have worked with them for some time, or been involved directly in their training.

Lack of regulation, professional closure and identity

As outlined earlier, the allied health workforce is heterogeneous, poorly defined and lacks systematic boundaries. Consequently, the support workforce associated with the allied health professions tends to be even more dispersed and fragmented than the allied health disciplines. The unifying features of allied health professional support workers are their lack of consistent formal training; heterogeneity of titles; diversity of roles and contexts; and range of employment conditions. While some discipline specific allied health support workers, such as occupational therapy assistants and physiotherapy assistants, may be eligible for associate membership of a professional body, a common complaint is the lack of clear definition or understanding of their role, which makes transferability difficult. Despite some exceptions, such as the closely defined role of physiotherapy assistant in the UK (Ellis and Connell 2001), formal training tends to be generic, supported by on-the-job, context and discipline specific development. Consequently, the role lacks a recognisable structure, even if it enables a more flexible and responsive workforce.

Generic vs discipline specific division of labour

A recent Australian model designed to introduce new allied health assistant roles had funding available for five generic roles. However, the positions were advertised as discipline specific roles (Nancarrow et al 2015). The managers responsible for the programme perceived that prospective allied health assistants would be more attracted to, and have a clearer understanding of, a discipline specific advertisement than a generic role title. This highlights that the contextually dependent nature of support worker skills means that there is a wide variety of views about their scope of practice, which is not helped by their lack of a clear regulatory framework. Thus, for example, a survey of podiatry assistants in the UK found their roles to vary from simple foot care for patients and clerical duties to a broader range of tasks, including assisting in nail and foot surgery (Farndon and Nancarrow 2003).

Supervision of the support workforce

A frequent point of contention for the allied health support workforce is the model of supervision. While there are broad assumptions that allied health support workers will work under the direct supervision of an allied health practitioner (Stute et al 2013), this does not always happen and is often not feasible. Supervision expectations tend to be derived from confusing lines of professional accountability, with allied health professionals assuming they are responsible for the outcomes of work delegated to support workers. As Nancarrow and Mackey (2005) relate, in relation to the occupational therapy assistant practitioner in Staffordshire in the UK where unregistered occupational therapists were unable to practice, the lack of a regulatory framework for them meant that a less qualified worker could perform largely similar tasks. Particular challenges to the supervision arrangements arise when the support worker is working with newly qualified allied health practitioners.

Conclusion

Understanding the support workforce associated with allied health professions in Australia and the UK is complicated by the diversity of professions that are incorporated within the allied health umbrella and the range of contexts and jurisdictions in which they work. The roles are further confounded by the increasing influence of the state and bureaucracies on the development of the support worker role, shifting tasks from a clear discipline specific division of labour to the ultimate 'boundary spanning role' taking on tasks delegated from multiple professions, delivering care in a range of settings, and working across different employer and jurisdictional boundaries. This approach contrasts with the typically more unified, neo–Weberian focus on the professional project, in which groups establish common goals and tasks and a common philosophy to achieve monopolisation (Saks 2010).

Where the medical, and to a certain extent nursing, professions have employed auxiliaries or delegated unwanted tasks within their division of labour, it has enabled the upward expansion of those professions into new areas of clinical specialisation. In contrast, rather than a professionalisation agenda, the driver for the growth of the allied health support workforce has predominantly been to increase service capacity at low cost, with little opportunity for upward expansion of skills of the allied health professions. Instead, such professions have largely moved into the narrower domains of their existing scope of practice, or taken on more managerial tasks such as assessment, training and supervision (Ellis and Connell 2001). One of the challenges facing the allied health professions is that, in the processes of 'ditching dirty work' (Hugman 1991) in times of high demand, they will find themselves unable to reclaim the territory in times of oversupply (Nancarrow and Borthwick 2005). Once these tasks have been relinquished to a wider workforce inhabited by new, non-specialist occupational groups, then, as demand rises, their scarcity value is likely to be reduced.

Increasingly, the codification and commodification of tasks has enabled the systematic transfer of roles between workers (Larson 1977). A suite of tools is emerging specifically to aid task disaggregation, re-engineering and re-allocation of roles based on service risks and needs (Smith and Duffy 2010) which could be seen to align with the Business Process Re-engineering outlined by McNulty and Ferlie (2004). More recently, technologies such as micro-credentialing have been introduced that support opportunities for the development of micro-specialisms, which include high volume, low risk tasks that can be undertaken by any appropriately credentialed worker (Nancarrow 2015). However in disaggregating tasks from a profession, the organising principles offered by a professional group may be lost (Adler et al 2008), as may the concept of shared professional identity or branding (Evetts 2006).

The interface between support workers and allied health professions are highly context dependent. In more highly structured and hierarchical hospital settings, allied health roles have been delegated to more junior staff on the ward and/or staff such as nurses delivering speech pathology or physiotherapy interventions on the wards who work more frequently with the patients. This in part comes about because of the way that allied health professions are employed. Since their skills tend to be nuanced and specialised around body parts or functions, allied health workers tend to work across a range of groups or wards, in a way that means that they identify issues and prescribe treatment, but may not be available to deliver treatment routines which are delegated. Nonetheless, the allied health support workforce is in transition. While it has provided opportunities for allied health professionals to expand their clinical reach by increasing the volume of service provision, the opportunities to expand upwards by broadening niche skills remain limited by historic relationships to the medical profession and their own internal hierarchies and restricted scale.

References

Abbott, A. (1981) 'Status and status strain in the professions', *American Journal of Sociology* 86(4): 819–35.

Adler, P.S., Kwon, S.-W. and Heckscher, C. (2008) 'Perspective – professional work: The emergence of collaborative community', *Organization Science* 19(2): 359–76.

Alaszewski, A. (1995) 'Restructuring health and welfare professions in the United Kingdom: The impact of internal markets on the medical, nursing and social work professions', in Johnson, T., Larkin, G. and Saks, M. (eds) *Health Professions and the State in Europe*, London: Routledge.

Allsop, J. (1995) 'Shifting spheres of opportunity: The professional powers of general practitioners within the British National Health Service', in Johnson, T., Larkin, G. and Saks, M. (eds) *Health Professions and the State in Europe*, London: Routledge.

Allsop, J. and Saks, M. (2002) 'Introduction: The regulation of the health professions', in Allsop, J. and Saks, M. (eds) *Regulating the Health Professions*, London: Sage.

Astley, J. (2000) 'Transforming allied health', *Australian Health Review* 23(4): 160–69.

Bach, S., Kessler, I. and Heron, P. (2008) 'Role redesign in a modernised NHS: The case of health care assistants', *Human Resource Management Journal* 18(2): 171–87.

Braverman, H. (1974) *Labor and Monopoly Capital*, New York: Monthly Review Press.

Buchan, J. and Dal Poz, M.R. (2002) 'Skill mix in the health care workforce: Reviewing the evidence', *Bulletin of the World Health Organization* 80(7): 575–80.

Carvalho, T. (2014) 'Changing connections between professionalism and managerialism: A case study of nursing in Portugal', *Journal of Professions and Organization* 1(2): 176–90.

Davies, C. (1995) *Gender and the Professional Predicament in Nursing*, New York: McGraw-Hill Education.

Dent, M., Chandler, J. and Barry, J. (eds) (2004) *Questioning the New Public Management*, Aldershot: Ashgate.

Department of Health (2000) *The NHS Plan: A Plan for Investment. A Plan for Reform*, London: The Stationery Office.

Ellis, B. and Connell, N. (2001) 'Factors determining the current use of physiotherapy assistants. Views on their future role in the South and West UK Region', *Physiotherapy* 87(2): 73–82.

England, K. and Dyck, I. (2011) 'Managing the body work of home care', *Sociology of Health and Illness* 33(2): 206–19.

Evetts, J. (2006) 'Short note: The sociology of professional groups: New directions', *Current Sociology* 54(1): 133–43.

Farndon, L. and Nancarrow, S. (2003) 'Employment and career development opportunities for podiatrists and foot care assistants in the NHS', *British Journal of Podiatry* 6(4): 103–108.

Foster, A. (2006) 'Assistant practitioners – context, purpose and opportunity', Assistant Practitioners: A one-day conference on the role of assistants in the team, London.

Freidson, E. (1970) *Profession of Medicine: A Study of the Sociology of Applied Knowledge*, New York: Dodd, Mead & Co.

Gilburt, H. (2016) *Supporting Integration through New Roles and Working across Boundaries*, London: King's Fund.

Ham, C. (1994) *Management and Competition in the New NHS*, Oxford: Radcliffe Medical Press.

Hancock, H., Campbell, S., Ramprogus, V. and Kilgour, J. (2005) 'Role development in health care assistants: The impact of education on practice', *Journal of Evaluation in Clinical Practice* 11(5): 489–98.

Hek, G., Singer, L. and Taylor, P. (2004) 'Cross-boundary working: A generic worker for older people in the community', *British Journal of Community Nursing* 9(6): 237–44.

Hugman, R. (1991) *Power in the Caring Professions*, Basingstoke: Macmillan.

Johnson, T. (2016) *Professions and Power*, Abingdon: Routledge Revivals.

Kessler, I. and Bach, S. (2007) *New Types of Worker Programme: Stage 1 Evaluation Report*, Leeds: Skills for Care.

Klein, R. (2013) *The New Politics of the NHS: From Creation to Reinvention*, 7th edition, London: Radcliffe Publishing,

Larkin, G. (1983) *Occupational Monopoly and Modern Medicine*, London: Tavistock.

Larkin, G. (1988) 'Medical dominance in Britain: Image and historical reality', *The Millbank Quarterly* 66(Supplement 2): 117–32.

Larkin, G. (1995) 'State control and the health professions in the United Kingdom', in Johnson, T., Larkin, G. and Saks, M. (eds) *Health Professions and the State in Europe*, London: Routledge.

Larkin, G. (2002) 'Regulating the professions allied to medicine', in Allsop, J. and Saks, M. (eds) *Regulating the Health Professions*, London: Sage.

Larson, M.S. (1977) *The Rise of Professionalism: A Sociological Analysis*, Berkeley, CA: University of California Press.

Le Cornu, K., Halliday, D., Swift, L., Ferris, L. and Gatiss, G. (2010) 'The current and future role of the dietetic support worker', *Journal of Human Nutrition and Dietetics* 23(3): 230–37.

Lecca, P.J., Valentine, P. and Lyons, K.J. (2003) *Allied Health: Practice Issues and Trends in the New Millennium*, London: Routledge.

Lizarondo, L., Kumar, S., Hyde, L. and Skidmore, D. (2010) 'Allied health assistants and what they do: A systematic review of the literature', *Journal of Multidisciplinary Healthcare* 3: 143.

Macdonald, K. (1995) *The Sociology of the Professions*, London: Sage.

Mackey, H. and Nancarrow, S.A. (2005) 'Assistant practitioners: Issues of accountability, delegation and competence', *International Journal of Therapy and Rehabilitation* 12(8).

Malin, N., Wilmot, S. and Manthorpe, J. (2002) *Key Concepts and Debates in Health and Social Policy*, Maidenhead: Open University Press.

McClimens, A., Nancarrow, S.A., Moran, A., Enderby, P. and Mitchell, C. (2010) '"Riding the bumpy seas": Or the impact of the knowledge skills framework component of the agenda for change initiative on staff in intermediate care settings', *Journal of Interprofessional Care* 24(1): 70–79.

McNulty, T. and Ferlie, E. (2004) 'Process transformation: Limitations to radical organizational change within public service organizations', *Organization Studies* 25(8): 1389–412.

Moran, A.M., Nancarrow, S.A., Wiseman, L., Maher, K., Boyce, R.A., Borthwick, A.M. and Murphy, K. (2012) 'Assisting role redesign: A qualitative evaluation of the implementation of a podiatry assistant role to a community health setting utilising a traineeship approach', *Journal of Foot and Ankle Research* 5(1): 30.

Nancarrow, S.A. (2004) 'Dynamic role boundaries in intermediate care services', *Journal of Interprofessional Care* 18(2): 141–51.

Nancarrow, S.A. (2015) 'Six principles to enhance health workforce flexibility', *Human Resources for Health* 13(1): 9.

Nancarrow, S.A. and Borthwick, A.M. (2005) 'Dynamic professional boundaries in the healthcare workforce', *Sociology of Health and Illness* 27(7): 897–919.

Nancarrow, S.A. and Mackey, H. (2005) 'The introduction and evaluation of an occupational therapy assistant practitioner', *Australian Occupational Therapy Journal* 52(4): 293–301.

Nancarrow, S.A., Moran, A. and Sullivan, R. (2015) 'Mechanisms for the effective implementation of an allied health assistant trainee: A qualitative study of a speech language pathology assistant', *Australian Health Review* 39(1): 101–108.

Nancarrow, S.A., Shuttleworth, P., Tongue, A. and Brown, L. (2005) 'Support workers in intermediate care', *Health and Social Care in the Community* 13(4): 338–44.

Nancarrow, S.A., Young, G., O'Callaghan, K., Jenkins, M., Philip, K. and Barlow, K. (2017) 'Shape of allied health: An environmental scan of 27 allied health professions in Victoria', *Australian Health Review* 41(3): 327–35.

NHS Modernisation Agency (2004) 'Introduction to role redesign and CWP', www.modern.nhs.uk/scripts/default.asp?site_id=65&id=21127

Noordegraaf, M. (2007) 'From "pure" to "hybrid" professionalism: Present-day professionalism in ambiguous public domains', *Administration and Society* 39(6): 761–85.

Olson, S. (2012) *Allied Health Workforce and Services: Workshop Summary*, Washington, DC: National Academies Press.

Ormandy, P., Long, A.F., Hulme, C.T. and Johnson, M. (2004) 'The role of the senior health care worker in critical care', *Nursing in Critical Care* 9(4): 151–8.

Ottosson, A. (2016) 'One history or many herstories? Gender politics and the history of physiotherapy's origins in the nineteenth and early twentieth century', *Women's History Review* 25(2): 296–319.

Pollock, A.M. (2004) *NHS plc: The Privatisation of Our Health Care*, London, Verso.

Pullenayegum, S., Fielding, B., Du Plessis, E. and Peate, I. (2005) 'The value of the role of the rehabilitation assistant', *British Journal of Nursing* 14(14): 778–84.

Robinson, A.J., McCall, M., DePalma, M.T., Clayton-Krasinski, D., Tingley, S., Simoncelli, S. and Harnish, L. (1994). 'Physical therapists' perceptions of the roles of the physical therapist assistant', *Physical Therapy* 74(6): 571–82.

Saks, M. (2010) 'Analyzing the professions: The case for the neo-Weberian approach', *Comparative Sociology* 9(6): 887–915.

Saks, M. (2015) *The Professions, State and the Market: Medicine in Britain, the United States and Russia*, Abingdon: Routledge.

Saks, M. (2016a) 'Professions and power: A review of theories of professions and power', in Dent, M., Bourgeault, I.L., Denis, J-L. and Kuhlmann, E. (eds) *The Routledge Companion to the Professions and Professionalism*, Abingdon: Routledge.

Saks, M. (2016b) 'The regulation of the English health professions: Zoos, circuses or safari parks?', in Liljegren, A. and Saks, M. (eds) *Professions and Metaphors: Understanding Professions in Society*, Abingdon: Routledge.

Saks, M. and Allsop, J. (2007) 'Social Policy, Professional Regulation and Health Support Work in the United Kingdom', *Social Policy and Society* 6(2): 165–77.

Salter, B. (2001) 'Who rules?: The new politics of medical regulation', *Social Science and Medicine* 52: 871–83.

Salvatori, P. (2001) 'The history of occupational therapy assistants in Canada: A comparison with the United States', *Canadian Journal of Occupational Therapy* 68(4): 217–27.

Shortell, S.M. (1974) 'Occupational prestige differences within the medical and allied health professions', *Social Science and Medicine* 8(1): 1–9.

Smith, R. and Duffy, J. (2010) 'Developing a competent and flexible workforce using the Calderdale Framework', *International Journal of Therapy and Rehabilitation* 17(5): 254–62.

Spilsbury, K. and Meyer, J. (2005) 'Making claims on nursing work: Exploring the work of healthcare assistants and the implications for registered nurses' roles', *Journal of Research in Nursing* 10(1): 65–83.

Stanmore, E., Ormrod, S. and Waterman, H. (2005) 'New roles in rehabilitation – the implications for nurses and other professionals', *Journal of Evaluation in Clinical Practice* 12(6): 656–64.

Stanmore, E. and Waterman, H. (2007) 'Crossing professional and organizational boundaries: The implementation of generic rehabilitation assistants within three organizations in the northwest of England', *Disability and Rehabilitation* 29(9): 751–59.

Strong, P. and Robinson, J. (1990) *The NHS: Under New Management*, Buckingham: Open University Press.

Stute, M., Hurwood, A., Hulcombe, J. and Kuipers, P. (2013) 'Defining the role and scope of practice of allied health assistants within Queensland public health services', *Australian Health Review* 37(5): 602–606.

Turnbull, C., Grimmer-Somers, K., Kumar, S., May, E., Law, D. and Ashworth, E. (2009) 'Allied, scientific and complementary health professionals: A new model for Australian allied health', *Australian Health Review* 33(1): 27–37.

Turner, B.S. (1985) 'Knowledge, skills and occupational strategy: The professionalisation of paramedical groups', *Community Health Studies* 9(1): 38–47.

Turner, B.S. (1995) *Medical Power and Social Knowledge*, 2nd edition, London: Sage.

Victorian Department of Health and Human Services (2016) *Allied Health Assistance Workforce Report: 55*, Melbourne: Victorian Government.

Wanless, D. (2002) *Securing Our Future Health: Taking a Long-Term View*, London: Stationery Office.

Webb, F., Farndon, L., Borthwick, A.M., Nancarrow, S.A. and Vernon, W. (2004) 'The development of support workers in allied health care: A case study of podiatry assistants', *British Journal of Podiatry* 7(3): 83–7.

Willis, E. (1983) *Medical Dominance: The Division of Labour in Australian Healthcare*, Sydney: George Allen and Unwin.

Zagrodney, K. and Saks, M. (2017) 'Personal support workers in Canada: The new precariat?', *Healthcare Policy* 13(2): 31–9.

SEVEN

Support workers in social care: Between social work professionals and service users

Andreas Liljegren, Anna Dunér and Elisabeth Olin

Introduction

In this chapter we shall explore the current debate about the role of support workers in social care – namely, whether they should be part of a service run by staff or users. The focus of the analysis is on two cases. The first is support services in group homes, which can be seen as a provider controlled. The second is personal assistance in domiciliary settings as a user-led service. The relative merits of formal training and the role of support services for disabled people, including people with various chronic health conditions, are discussed against a wider context of user preferences in a situation where, as in other international contexts, politicians are seeking cost savings and hold the key to future developments.

When professions came into the spotlight with authors like Freidson (1970) and Larson (1977), a few top professions like medicine were described and analysed using the metaphor of hierarchy (Liljegren 2016). The focus at that point was on how these top professions act to remain in the upper part of the hierarchy – as, for example, through the use of 'market shelters' (Freidson 2001). The neo-Weberian perspective was created as a counter to more naïve perspectives that only highlighted the virtues of professionalism (Saks 2010). The claim on power within society for professions based on credentialism and formal knowledge can be seen as the basis of professional power (Collins 1979; Liljegren et al 2014). In this perspective educational facilities, including universities, are both the producers of formal knowledge and responsible for introducing and socialising new members into the ideology of professions – such that, for example, formal knowledge should be rewarded economically, symbolically and socially.

Within contemporary research on professions there is increased interest in broadening the discussion, taking into account occupational and other groups that are not traditionally cast as professions or semi-professions – including laypersons (Liljegren et al 2017), service users (Eyal 2013) and support workers (Dunér and Olin 2011; Saks 1995; Zagrodney and Saks 2017). These groups might not be defined as professions, but can still be described as having expertise in the sense that they make claims on getting the work done better (Eyal 2013). However, against this, support workers *per se* have been described as belonging to a new precariat as they have a weak position in the labour market, with low salaries, poor opportunities for advancement, low job insecurity and few full-time employment opportunities (Zagrodney and Saks 2017).

For more traditional professionals, a higher degree of autonomy can be expected, not least because they have been better organised in initiating their own professionalisation. In contrast, the new precariat of support workers can be expected to have weaker organisations that speak on their behalf (or none at all), such as general unions that also organise other, even competing, occupational groups. Auxiliary workers are also to a lesser degree based on technical skills and to a higher degree on everyday knowledge and, for that reason, have a much weaker jurisdiction. In the case of support workers in social care, the jurisdiction is not threatened by traditional professional groups like social workers or nurses as the support workers do a form of 'dirty work' (Hughes 1963). Instead the challenge to their jurisdiction comes from users claiming that they have the expertise to make the decisions on how to organise services. In that way it is a much more open question if, when, where and how these groups can and should be professionalised with different demands coming from above (the state or higher positioned occupational groups), within (their own claims) or below (as service users).

As previously indicated, the aim of the paper – against this backcloth – is to describe and analyse the role of support workers for disabled people in two settings, support workers in residential social care and so-called personal assistants in domiciliary care, both operating in Swedish social work. These two settings have chosen radically different ways to organise social care in terms of power relations. First, however, we outline the general socio-political context that prevails in Sweden.

Swedish welfare policies

Sweden is regarded as a universal welfare state in terms of its systems of benefits and services linked to the lifetime needs of its citizens

(Esping-Andersen 1990). The formal goals of the Swedish welfare system comprise universalism and extensive coverage, although a policy shift has taken place towards more individualised care and services with an emphasis on consumer choice. Since 1992 the local authorities in its 290 self-governed municipalities have overall responsibility for social care and services for older people as well as for disabled people, including in residential care settings as defined by a Swedish Government Bill of 1990/91.

However, the division of responsibility for health care is complex and varies depending on local agreements (Edgren and Stenberg 2006). Health care is provided by both county councils/regions and municipalities. The county councils are responsible for all health care except for older or disabled people living in residential settings. Within the county councils the regional/local hospitals are responsible for acute medical care that requires hospital admission, and primary health care centres are responsible for outpatient care. Municipal health care provides for those living in residential settings and, after local agreements, for home nursing for those living in their own homes as well. In addition, the responsibility for personal assistance, according to the Act Concerning Support and Services to Persons with Certain Functional Impairments, is shared between the national Swedish Social Insurance Agency (SSIA) and the local municipal authorities. The SSIA is responsible for providing assistance allowance to users requiring over 20 hours personal assistance with 'basic needs' each week. Local authorities are responsible for providing personal assistance to users in domiciliary settings with less extensive requirements.

Swedish social work in this context can be described as a highly academic field of work and is dominated by university trained professionals with a degree in social work. Often this group is employed in social welfare departments, primarily with qualified needs–assessment and decision making or relational and motivational work connected to different kinds of treatments. Thus, the assessments and decisions of social workers at both local and national levels guide the provision of services by support workers to disabled people. The main tasks of the auxiliary social workers are to provide support in everyday living, including personal hygiene, household chores and social and cultural activities. Support workers in group homes, or other traditional residential support services, are often seen as requiring a non–academic basic education. For employment as a personal assistant, though, no formal training is required.

Support services for disabled people are among the biggest areas of employment in Sweden. In 2016 72,566 people were employed as personal assistants and 61,640 people were employed to provide caring services in other support services for disabled people, including in group homes (SCB 2017). The majority of personal assistants are employed in the private sector, many of them work part time, and their employment is tied to the needs of the assistant user which often means inconvenient working hours. Support workers in group homes are mostly employed by municipal authorities. They often have possibilities to work full time and have more regulated working schedules as compared to personal assistants. Thus, support workers in group homes have more secure and regulated working conditions than personal assistants. The work of personal assistants might include heavy lifting on their own and working a few hours in the morning and a few in the evening when the service users need more assistance.

Professional vs user-controlled services

Normalisation and integration have been the ideological guiding principles of Swedish disability policy from the late 1960s. However, during the 1980s, welfare services for disabled people were criticised, both in Sweden and in other countries. One of the most dynamic actors in this debate was the Independent Living Movement, which criticised the philosophy of normalisation and integration for neglecting the barriers to, as well as the discrimination against, disabled people in society. This criticism also included the paternalistic provision of services, both in relation to formal services in institutional settings and informal care from families (Pearson et al 2014).

Instead, the Independent Living Movement, and other organisations of disabled people, called for user-led services characterised by choice and control by disabled people themselves. This led to a fundamental shift in the distribution of power between user and provider. They claimed that it is the user who is the expert, not the staff, and that they have the competence to determine how the work should be performed (Dunér and Olin 2017; Egard 2011; Morris 2004; Ratzka 1996; Shakespeare 2014; White et al 2010). They emphasised disabled people's right to independent living and opposed traditional views of disabled people as 'medical cases' or 'objects of charity and care' or 'objects of pity and (over)protection'. Professional power, family care and emotional involvement were thus rejected.

In Sweden a paradigm shift came in 1994 when the Act Concerning Support and Services to Persons with Certain Functional Impairments came into force. The intention was to advance individual rights, self-determination and participation in society for disabled people with comprehensive and lasting support needs (SGOR 2008). The Act provides strengthened support rights for particular groups of disabled people, in addition to what they may receive through other legislation, including the right to individual services such as personal assistance and collectivistic support services in group homes. Thus, the state intervened indirectly by strengthening the weaker party in relation to welfare organisations, which meant a shift in the power balance between users and the providers of support (Barron et al 2000). The intention to advance the self-determination and participation of disabled people in society encompasses all individuals covered by the law, regardless of which type of support they receive – either personal assistance or other support services as in group homes.

It should be noted that the move from emphasising individual control and self- determination, to downplaying collective forms of support, can be seen as 'time typical' as it reflects wider societal changes and trends. Thus, striving for personalisation, in both law and policy, is not only a shift away from paternalistic provision of services towards user control, but is also linked to a broader consumerist discourse, emphasising individual freedom of choice in the market (Brennan et al 2017; Pearson et al 2014). However, it has been argued that it is important to problematise the consumerist assumption of rational, well-informed and competent consumers, and take into account the diversity of disabled people. Neglecting to do so may result in inequality of opportunities among disabled people (Askheim 2003; Askheim et al 2013; Brennan et al 2016; Olin and Dunér 2016). In recent years, much of the debate about support services for disabled people has focused on the so-called 'cost-problem' associated with personal assistance, and politicians have pointed to the necessity of cost savings (Westerberg 2017). Group homes have once again emerged as the preferred alternative, especially for disabled people with complex needs and/or learning difficulties (NBHW 2017; Westerberg 2017).

Two empirical cases: social support workers in residential care and personal assistants in domiciliary care

Empirical data from two earlier studies will be used to illustrate the discussion. The first study (Dunér and Olin 2011) focused on how support workers from local municipal social care viewed their professional role and what competence they thought was needed to perform their work. Participants were seven support workers, six women and one man, who had between four and 25 years of experience within their profession. Five participants had a degree in social care, one was an educationalist, one had a degree in social science from a university college, and several also had supplementary courses from vocational colleges or supplementary university courses. An official responsible for development issues in a municipality divided into ten local authorities was helpful in recruiting participants to the study. The group met on two occasions for about two and a half hours each time. The researchers acted as moderators, and the discussions were guided by a thematic interview guide. At the meetings, much room was given to the participants' own reflections.

The second study (Dunér and Olin 2017; Olin and Dunér 2016) focused on the personal assistance provided by one or several family members of the user. It was based on qualitative interviews with users of personal assistance and family members employed as personal assistants. Participants were recruited through user organisations, an internet forum in which disability-related issues were discussed, and recommendations from our first participants in snowball fashion (Lee 1993). In total 40 persons participated: 17 users of personal assistance and 23 family members (partners, sons or daughters, parents, or siblings) employed as personal assistants. The interviews lasted between 45 to 90 minutes, with varied settings chosen by the participants, including a room at the university, their homes and workplaces. Two of the interviews were conducted via the telephone. A thematic interview guide was used. The interviews were open ended, allowing the interviewees to speak freely and the researchers to follow up on emerging themes.

Case 1: Social support workers in residential care

Residential care for disabled people is organised in a traditional way where profession/support workers have a strong position in relation to the service users as experts, with their conception of needs and legitimacy deriving from their formal training. This case can be seen as a setting which is striving for more professionally oriented social care. The staff in group homes for disabled people had a superior power position in relation to the residents. Sometimes professional power was used to limit the possibilities of the residents to control and self-determine their everyday life. However, the staff could also use their power to guide and support the residents into social relationships and activities outside the group home. For some residents, guidance and support from staff could be a prerequisite for increased independence and participation in society. However, there is also a risk that staff define their task as training disabled people in social skills and thus enforce their own socially accepted norms on the residents. To require higher education for staff in group homes is a controversial issue, as some see it as threatening the self-determination and control of users. Nonetheless, studies show that staff with academic education may be more responsive to the needs and wishes of users, and decrease the risk of violence and oppression (see, for example, Ahnlund 2008).

It has been demonstrated that over the past decades that the position of the social work profession has remained the same, even though the focus of the staff has changed in accordance with the ideological changes in disability policies from a collectivist to a more individualistic view (Olin 2003). During the 'collective era', the job was organised and performed in relation to the entire resident group, but today staff are supposed to organise and adapt their work according to the needs and wishes of each individual. In the focus group interviews the informants claimed that the complexity of the work demands well-educated staff. One informant claimed that the ideal education would be:

> a basic education as 'support assistant', with a pedagogical focus on different disabilities and impairments.

However, there are no formal requirements concerning education to work in group homes. Employers have made several attempts, both at a local and a national level, to increase the amount of academically-trained staff but so far without great success. The solution has been to offer working tasks and salaries good enough to attract such staff. This means that support workers at group homes have various educational levels and consequently different denominations and competencies. In the focus group interviews, there were divergent opinions about the value of well-trained staff. Some of the informants saw the advantages of formal training:

> 'Where I work, my boss has employed staff who have at least vocational education. It's an incredible improvement compared with my former working place.'

But others felt that an excessive level of education may result in the scientific perspective taking precedence over the human one:

> 'Then they came from this work group and it became very scientific. They sat and talked and talked and the user sat next to them. Then we forget that we work with people. It became too scientific because they had an academic education.'

Nonetheless, today's work in group homes also includes a requirement for administrative competence, as increasing emphasis is put on written documentation of their work. Mansell and Elliot (2001) show that administrative tasks are defined as having the highest priority and status. According to the informants, different kinds of social documentation were essential tools to ensure their quality of work and to visualise its complexity. Some informants were very clear that what is not documented does not exist:

> 'But if nothing is documented, we have nothing to go through. How is independent development for this person? I cannot read anything about it.'

In parallel, a discussion emerged in the focus groups about the character of the support provided. The informants viewed the importance of care in different ways. Some felt that care was linked to an 'old-time' disability ideology, where disabled people were regarded as passive and dependent, in need of protection. They emphasised the need for the agency of disabled people and the performance of instrumental tasks. But there were also voices highlighting the importance of personal relationships and emotional involvement between staff and residents, often associated with caring, even if it could have complications:

> 'You can be personal, but you do not have to tell your whole family history. One can be a confidant, but it's really hard to set the limit for what's too private.'

Some of the informants preferred not to be emotionally engaged and exchangeability was one way to do it.

> 'It's the schedule that controls the activity. I can go inside and shower someone even though I did not meet that person during the evening. It is the situation that governs, not me as a person.'

This was also related to the dilemma between defining the group home as the residents' private home or a workplace for the staff. The former definition is associated with an individual orientation, emotional engagement and flexibility, while a workplace is associated with a collective orientation, distance and formal rules (Olin 2003). When it came to the possibility for residents to steer and control support, a complex picture appeared. On the one hand, it seemed that they had very limited opportunities to decide what to do, when and with whom:

> 'We have scheduled staff time for one hour a week, when the residents themselves choose what they want to do.'

Some of the group homes had very strict routines which, maybe due to low staffing, obviously making it difficult for the residents to control their support services and their everyday life. This way to organise the job has great similarities with the era when disabled people living in group homes were treated as a collective, not as individuals:

> 'We have scheduled different days for different activities. We are six staff for six residents, so if some residents put pressure on the routines it affects the other residents too. So if someone does not want to shower when it is planned, then the person has to wait three days for next time.'

On the other hand there were also informants that reflected the importance for residents to have access to relationships and community outside the group home. Here self-determination was not exclusively associated with the individuals' own choice, but regarded as a process arising in social relations with the staff. The importance of the responsibility of, and initiative from, the staff was stressed:

> 'I believe that we must take our responsibility, that we must be the one that helps to convey social relations. They [the residents] may not have, or take, the initiative to seek other networks or social relationships outside the group home.'

In sum, in the case of residential care the reflections from support workers are about, on the one hand, how the professional domain should be interpreted by an occupational group based on formal education and following strict routines focused on administrative documentation and, on the other, how it can be seen through the lens of a more personal and flexible ideology centred less on formal education.

Case 2: Personal assistants in domiciliary care

Personal assistance in domiciliary settings has formed the basis of an alternative model for support services. This case can be seen as an example of user-oriented social care. Personal assistance means that users exercise the maximum control over how services are organised and performed. One key goal with personal assistants is to achieve equal rights, equal opportunities and self-determination – independent living – for disabled people. This case can be seen as based on a user perspective where the user dominates the care setting. Simply put, personal assistance means that the user is 'the boss' (Ratzka 1996). In one of the interviews, a user pointed to the importance of the unique needs and preferences in shaping the assistance:

'Personal assistance is unique, no-one has the same preferences as I do, and thus no-one has the same way of supervising the work as I have. I compromise and adapt to things that other people would not.'

Thus, individual users must have the opportunity to recruit, train, schedule and supervise their own assistants. One of the assistance users expressed how she looked on her twofold roles as both user and employer:

'I'm responsible for the working environment of the assistants, so that they can get on and have clear directives. My assistants shouldn't talk about working conditions with me when they work as assistants, then I'm just Susanna, not their employer. If they want to discuss such issues they have to e-mail me and I can choose when I answer them, and we can make an appointment to discuss further. To separate a bit ...'

She also continues to emphasise that personal assistance means that she is in total control of the situation. Thus, the role of her personal assistants is to carry out instrumental tasks without emotional involvement (see also Shakespeare 2014):

'When we are outdoors, my assistants walk one or two metres behind me. In the car it's silence if I don't talk to them. Now when the assistant handed you the water, and you thanked her, she didn't say anything. In our world it was me who gave you the water and thus it would have been odd if she would respond "you're welcome".'

However, being the boss means that the assistance user needs to perform extensive work, as well as to take on responsibilities for the work situation of users. As another of the interviewed assistance users explained:

> 'It's like being a boss 24 hours a day and not being able to go home. It's tough ... So, it's tough and I still think it is. You're supposed to think about working environment, that the assistant should have time to eat and everything ...'

As disabled people were expected to take on roles as experts and managers of their own assistance, and assumed to oppose professional interference in their lives, no formal training is needed, or even wanted, for the personal assistants. Instead, many user organisations, supporting the Independent Living ideology, arrange training for users in order to learn the skills of managing their personal assistance (Egard 2011). One of the interviewed users explained the process of learning to supervise her assistants, according to her own preferences as well as the needs of the assistants:

> 'Well, I think I have a much more explicit approach to myself and to my assistants today than I had ten or fifteen years back when the assistance started. Now I can be very clear about what's OK and what's not. But some assistants are more self-going than others. Some need a lot of support and guidance, practical instructions and so forth.'

Most users found the task of instructing their personal assistants simple:

> 'It's hard to explain to a stranger. You can say "put on the sock on the right foot first". Equally "... damn", the next time they start with the left foot.'

However, in some cases the situation might be more complex – for example, for users who require not only practical support with everyday tasks, but also support with communication, decision making and/or directing their personal assistance. One of the parents we interviewed reflects:

> 'There needs to be someone who sees the whole picture and makes everything work. Maybe it's not enough with only personal assistants when you can't speak for yourself, when you have to rely on others' ability to interpret your

needs and preferences. If you can speak for yourself, relatives don't need to be involved in the same way, I think.'

Here the personal assistant may need skills developed in order to take charge of the situation and be responsive to the needs and wishes of the user (Ahnlund 2008).

To sum up, according to the Independent Living ideology the users are the experts on their support services, and are thus the ones to decide who they want to hire as their assistant, determine what chores they want them to do and supervise how the assistance is performed. If there is a need for formal training, it is the user who should get it, so that they in their turn can train their assistants. However, in our interviews, a more complex picture emerged, especially for service users who needed support to be in control of their support services and their everyday life.

Discussion: whither professionalisation?

There is no given way as to how support workers should relate to their users, but most often it seems as if they have successfully made claims on a more dominant position with the final say on many issues. However, the two cases described have gone in different directions in terms of the power balance between auxiliary social workers and the service user. From earlier research we have noted that there are cases where user groups support the profession in alliance with professionals supporting and promoting the interests of a specific client group (Eyal 2013). What we see in the case of users in relation to Swedish support workers is a bifurcation of positions.

Support workers within residential care have taken a traditional stand. They have the necessary expertise and the service users are subordinated by supplementary social workers. In this case the staff discussed the pros and cons of professionalism – such as the relative merits of professional training and formal knowledge. With varying degrees of success, they negotiated about the exact boundaries of user/ professional jurisdiction or, in more practical terms, on who should decide what, when, where and why. However, the staff still held a stronger position. What is argued for here is professionalisation in terms of increased formal education. Nonetheless, when support workers in this setting reflect on their role within the organisation and in relation to service users, they do so more as a bureaucrat than a professional with administrative skills, following strict routines to relate to users in a detached way instead of trying to build more personal relationships.

This is not what is traditionally connected to professionalism in social work, which is based on strong relations with service users being more flexible using their own discretion.

These strivings for a more bureaucratic form of work focusing on administrative documentation and following strict routines in social work can in fact be seen as a form of deprofessionalisation of the Swedish support workers as formal knowledge is used to turn the support workers into bureaucrats instead of professionals, where being more professional is interpreted as being more personal and flexible. However, according to the Independent Living ideology, which may be imposed or inflicted on personal assistants in domiciliary care, the users are the experts on their support services. If there is a need for formal training, it is the users who should receive it, so that they in turn can train their assistants. This can be seen as a case of the service users subordinating the support workers. So key questions are: what content should formal education take and for whom? and what are the implications for professionalisation?

It has been argued that attempts to increase professionalisation in support services for disabled people risks strengthening the power of support workers and, accordingly, lessens the power of users (Eliasson 1992; Lindqvist 2007; Wearness 1984). According to this line of argument, welfare arrangements are often characterised by an emphasis on the perspective of the support workers and a resulting lack of attention to the intentions and agency of disabled people (Morris 2004; Oliver 1990; White et al 2010). Inherent in traditional support services is their hierarchical structure with the user at the bottom. Thus, demands have been raised from a user perspective, instead of a paternalistic and professional perspective, taking the power balance between the support workers and the users into consideration. There is therefore a related challenge for professional social services to balance the right of choice and control of disabled people, with reasonable working conditions for support workers. The needs assessments and decisions of professional social workers are thus of vital importance, as they guide the support workers in their provision of services. Therefore, professional social workers have to take into account the diversity of disabled people and use their professional power either to enable service users to determine how the work is to be performed or to secure service users' needs for support in order to create good living conditions.

From a theoretical perspective these cases are about professionalisation from above (the state), from within (their own claims) or deprofessionalisation from below (the clients). At a time when the

New Public Management and reducing costs are important in all issues involving the welfare sector in Sweden we suspect that more cost-effective residential care will be prioritised. Our interpretation of the kind of ideas suggested for staff in residential care is that it is in line with the organisational professionalism described by Evetts (2009), where staff might take the interest of the organisation instead of the service users (see also Liljegren 2012; Liljegren and Parding 2010; Parding and Liljegren 2016). Support workers can be seen as being squeezed between, on the one hand, an organisation that makes demands following strict rules and budgetary constraints and, on the other, a situation where service users make demands that they are the experts and should be the focus – thus professionalising the service user in the sense that they receive the formal education and not the staff. Both of these paths might end up in them becoming the new precariat of social care, along with personal assistants in domiciliary care (see also Chapter two which explores related conceptions of the precariat).

Conclusion

We conclude by suggesting what steps might be taken to avoid this polarised situation. If we are to follow in the footsteps of one of the sociology of professions' most interesting writers, Freidson (2001), he would probably say that we have three alternative ways to deal with the situation where both residential and domiciliary support workers end up in precarious situations: bureaucracy, market solutions or professionalism. Each of these situations will now be briefly explored.

We are rather pessimistic about the possibilities posed by bureaucracy and the market. The bureaucratic aspects will always be an important part of social work, both in Sweden and internationally, but locally-run bureaucracies led by local politicians have a tendency to take the interest of the organisation rather than the citizen moving towards organisational professionalism, as described. Both the organisation and local politicians in the era of the New Public Management have focused ever more on staying on track economically. This is simply seen as a strategy for survival in order to stay in office. Stronger market solutions will probably not be a helpful way either. The economic gains from giving support workers, say, three hours of work in the morning and three in the afternoon and letting the salaries stay low are just too great. So would professionalism solve this? If we see professionalisation as originating from the professions themselves (from within), it is unlikely that such professional groups as nurses and social workers will make a strong case for better working conditions for support workers. It is very rare that a more highly positioned group in a power hierarchy does so, regardless of social context. It seems as if all the powerful actors have strong interests in letting support workers stay in a precarious situation.

In our view, the only realistic option would be professionalisation from above, letting politicians at the national level set standards for education and working conditions for support workers. However, it should not be taken for granted that this kind of precarious employment is seen as negative politically. In the Swedish context it has been argued that more employment with low qualifications is needed because it is the only option for some groups such as immigrants. This argument has been put forward by both liberal and right-wing parties in Sweden. Against this, the Swedish labour unions and the Social Democratic Party claim that jobs with low salaries are not the appropriate way forward. They prefer to increase the training for these groups to enhance their attractiveness on the labour market. So, to conclude, there are many winners in allowing support workers in residential and domiciliary care to stay in a precarious situation – and an initiative to change this would probably have to come from national politics, if there is an interest in so doing. This question of political will is a familiar dilemma in policy making about support work internationally.

References

Ahnlund, P. (2008) *Omsorg som arbete. Om utbildning, arbetsmiljö och relationer i äldre- och handikappomsorgen*, Umeå: Umeå University.

Askheim, O. (2003) 'Personal assistance for people with intellectual impairments: Experiences and dilemmas', *Disability and Society* 18(3): 325–39.

Askheim, O., Amdersen, J., Guldvik, I. and Johansen, V. (2013) 'Personal assistance: What happens to the arrangement when the number of users increases and new user groups are included?', *Disability and Society* 28(3): 353–66.

Barron, K., Michailakis, D. and Söder, M. (2000) 'Funktionshindrade och den offentliga hjälpapparaten', in Szebehely, M. and Barron, K. (eds) *Välfärd, vård och omsorg*, Stockholm: Fritzes Offentliga Publikationer.

Brennan, C., Rice, J., Traustadottir, R. and Anderberg, P. (2017) 'How can states ensure access to personal assistance when service delivery is decentralized? A multi-level analysis of Iceland, Norway and Sweden', *Scandinavian Journal of Disability Research* 19(4): 334–46.

Brennan, C., Traustadottir, R., Rice, J. and Anderberg, P. (2016) 'Negotiating independence, choice and autonomy: Experiences of parents who coordinate personal assistance on behalf of their adult son or daughter', *Disability and Society* 31(5): 604–21.

Collins, R. (1979) *The Credential Society: An Historical Sociology of Education and Stratification*, New York: Academic Press.

Dunér, A. and Olin, E. (2011) En begynnande professionalisering? Om gränsarbete och kompetenskrav inom funktionshinderverksamhet och äldreomsorg', *Socialvetenskaplig Tidskrift* 18(4): 336–53.

Dunér, A. and Olin, E. (2017) 'Personal assistance from family members as an unwanted situation, an optimal solution or an additional good? The Swedish example', *Disability and Society* 33(1): 1–19.

Edgren, L. and Stenberg, G. (2006) *Närsjukvårdens ansikten*, Lund: Studentlitteratur.

Egard, H. (2011) *Personlig assistans i praktiken- beredskap, initiativ och vänskaplighet,* Lund: Lund University.

Eliasson, R. (1992) 'Omsorg som lönearbete: Om Taylorisering och professionalisering', in Eliasson, R. (ed) *Egenheter och allmänheter. En antologi om omsorg och omsorgens villkor,* Lund: Arkiv Förlag.

Esping-Andersen G. (1990) *The Three Worlds of Welfare Capitalism*, Cambridge: Cambridge University Press.

Evetts, J. (2009) 'New professionalism and New Public Management: Changes, continuities and consequences', *Comparative Sociology* 2: 247–66.

Eyal, G. (2013) 'For a sociology of expertise: The social origins of the autism epidemic', *American Journal of Sociology* 118(4): 863–907.

Freidson, E. (1970) *Profession of Medicine: A Study of the Sociology of Applied Knowledge*, New York: Dodd, Mead & Co.

Freidson, E. (2001) *Professionalism: The Third Logic*, Chicago, IL: University of Chicago Press.

Hughes, E.C. (1963) 'Professions', *Daedalus 92*(4): 655–68.

Larson, M.S. (1977) *The Rise of Professionalism: A Sociological Analysis*, Berkeley: California University Press.

Lee, R.M. (1993) *Doing Research on Sensitive Topics*, Thousand Oaks, CA: Sage.

Liljegren, A. (2012) 'Pragmatic professionalism: Micro level discourse in social work', *European Journal of Social Work* 15(3): 295–312.

Liljegren, A. (2016) 'Key metaphors in the sociology of professions: Occupations as hierarchies and landscapes', in Liljegren, A. and Saks, M. (eds) *Professions and Metaphors: Understanding Professions in Society*, London: Routledge.

Liljegren, A., Höjer, S. and Forkby, T. (2014) 'Laypersons, professions and governance in the welfare state: The Swedish child protection system', *Professions and Organization* 1: 161–75.

Liljegren, A., Höjer, S. and Forkby, T. (2017) '"I don't want to tell you how to do your job, but …" Layperson challenging the authority of professionals in Swedish child protection', *Nordic Social Work Research* 8: 50–63.

Liljegren, A. and Parding, K. (2010) 'Ändrad styrning av välfärdsprofessioner: Exemplet evidensbasering i socialt arbete', *Socialvetenskaplig Tidskrift* 3–4: 270–88.

Lindqvist, R. (2007) *Funktionshindrade i välfärdssamhället*, Malmö: Gleerup.

Mansell, J. and Elliot, E. (2001) 'Staff members prediction of consequences for their work in residential settings', *American Journal on Mental Retardation* 106(5): 434–47.

Morris, J. (2004) 'Independent living and community care: A disempowering framework', *Disability and Society* 19(5): 427–42.

NBHW (2017) *Insatser och stöd till personer med funktionsnedsättning – Lägesrapport 2017*, Stockholm: Socialstyrelsen.

Olin, E. (2003) *Uppbrott och förändring. När ungdomar med utvecklingsstörning flyttar hemifrån*, Gothenburg: Department of Social Work, University of Gothenburg.

Olin, E. and Dunér, A. (2016) 'A matter of love and labour? Parents working as personal assistants for their adult disabled children', *Nordic Social Work Research* 6(1): 38–52.

Oliver, M. (1990) *The Politics of Disablement*, London: MacMillan.

Parding, K. and Liljegren, A. (2016) 'Individual development plans as governance tools: Changed governance of teachers' work', *Scandinavian Journal of Educational Research* 61(6): 698–700.

Pearson, C., Ridley, J. and Hunter, S. (2014) *Self-Directed Support: Personalisation, Choice and Control*, Edinburgh: Dunedin Academic Press.

Ratzka, A. (1996) *Introduction to Direct Payments for Personal Assistance*, Farsta: Independent Living Institute.

Saks, M. (1995) *Professions and the Public Interest: Medical Power, Altruism and Alternative Medicine*, London: Routledge.

Saks, M. (2010) 'Analyzing the professions: The case for the neo-Weberian approach', *Comparative Sociology* 9(6): 887–915.

SCB (2017) 'De 20 vanligaste yrkena för kvinnor', www.scb.se/hitta-statistik/statistik-efter-amne/arbetsmarknad/sysselsattning-forvarvsarbete-och-arbetstider/yrkesregistret-med-yrkesstatistik/pong/tabell-och-diagram/20-vanligaste-yrkena-for-kvinnor/

SGOR (2008) *Möjlighet att leva som andra Ny lag om stöd och service till vissa personer med funktionsnedsättning*, Stockholm: Fritzes.

Shakespeare, T. (2014) *Disability Rights and Wrongs Revisited*, London: Routledge.

Wearness, K. (1984) 'The rationality of caring', *Economic and Industrial Democracy* 5: 185–211.

Westerberg, B. (2017) *Personlig assistans – en kritisk granskning av regeringens direktiv till LSSutredningen*, Stockholm: Westerberg, B.

White, G., Lloyd Sipson, J., Gonda, C., Ravesloot, C. and Coble, Z. (2010) 'Moving from independence to interdependence: A conceptual model of better understanding community participation of centers for Independent Living Consumers', *Journal of Disability Policy Studies* 20(4): 233–40.

Zagrodney, K. and Saks, M. (2017) 'Personal support workers in Canada: The new precariat?', *Healthcare Policy 13*(2): 31–9.

EIGHT

Health professionals and peer support workers in mental health settings

Aukje Leemeijer and Mirko Noordegraaf

Introduction

In the past 20 years, a new kind of health support worker has emerged in Western mental health care, the so-called 'peer support worker' (Hurley et al 2016; Mowbray et al 1996; Repper and Carter 2011). Peer support workers are former mental health care clients, who use their client experience to support other users of mental health care during their recovery process. Peer support workers' unique asset is their 'experiential knowledge', which they add to the delivery of mental health services. Although this sounds reasonable and relevant, and although the rise of peer support workers is clearly visible throughout mental health care, from the neo-Weberian perspective adopted in this chapter this rise is not without questions and is not uncontested. In fact, peer support workers seem to be struggling. This is related to the complexities of forming a new occupation (Abbott 1988; McMurray 2010; Tholen 2017), especially when workers must position themselves vis-à-vis existing professionals like psychiatrists, psychologists and nurses. In addition, it is related to the complexities of using and *incorporating* experiential knowledge, especially when expert knowledge and evidence are privileged.

In this chapter we will focus on the rise and role of peer support workers in mental health care in The Netherlands. We describe how the emergence of peer support workers is taking place, what kind of development they go through, and how relationships between this new type of worker and regular mental health professionals takes shape. We analyse this development from the perspective of generic professionalisation theory, but we use findings from a specific recent study on peer support workers, and we analyse the way in which expertise, evidence and experiences are interwoven – or not. In this way we can examine the potential incorporation of peer support workers in mental health care teams, in terms of both *control* and *content*, as professionalisation is a matter of establishing 'controlled content' (Noordegraaf 2007). We examine how they position themselves and are taken seriously (control), as well as how their expertise, that is experiences, are linked to the services rendered (content).

Peer support workers in mental health care

The objective to enhance *client centredness* has been an important development in mental health care in Western countries (Baklien and Bongaardt 2014). This is driven by a variety of developments, which can also be seen in the broader field of health care. The introduction of *marketisation* in health care, since the end of last century, has stimulated a stronger orientation towards clients' wishes, goals and perspectives. Many forms of client participation in the development, execution and evaluation of care have arisen to ensure higher appreciation by clients, supposedly resulting in more clients and higher production rates. Another, more normative, reason to enhance client centredness has its roots in the *democratisation* and *emancipation* movements of the 1960s and 1970s. Since then, the idea of 'nothing about us without us' – a mantra from the disability rights movement – has fuelled the efforts of clients and their representative organisations to gain more influence.

As a result, in the 1970s and the following decades, client peer groups, self-help groups and consumer-run drop-in and activity centres emerged as an alternative for the existing mental health care services (Baklien and Bongaardt 2014; Dixon et al 1994; Mowbray et al 1996). Within these settings and as a result of sharing client experiences, new insights developed about the meaning of 'recovery'. Recovery was defined more broadly than just recovery in a medical sense, now also including emotional and social recovery and the capability to live a meaningful and fulfilling life despite one's psychiatric problems (Boevink 2017; Boertien et al 2012; Hunt and Resnick 2015). In addition, 'consumers' of mental health care took up roles as peer mentor or peer support, using their client experience to help fellow sufferers of psychiatric illness.

Gradually, these approaches and insights found their way into existing mental health care institutions (Baklien and Bongaardt 2014; Fisk et al 2000; Hunt and Resnick 2015). Peer mentor roles previously at the fringes of health care institutions transformed into more formal roles, with mentors now participating in the execution of mental health services. Clients and former clients were introduced as *'experts by experience*', engaged in formal service delivery and recognised as valuable contributors to the recovery process of people suffering from psychiatric problems (Dixon et al 1994; Gates and Akabas 2007; Repper and Carter 2011). In order to help clients use their client experiences to support others, client organisations and educational institutions developed training courses and education programmes. Initially these 'experts by experience' took on the role of volunteers in client initiatives and mental health institutions. They supported clients in peer groups, provided information for clients and their family, and/ or shared their stories with professionals to enhance their awareness of what it means to suffer from psychiatric problems and to receive treatment. Over time their roles transformed into more formal ones and are now developing towards a new occupation in mental health care. During the past 20 years many health care institutions in Western countries (especially in Anglo-Saxon countries and Northern and Western Europe) employ so-called peer support workers as visible and paid members of professional teams in formal service delivery (Repper and Carter 2011). In most cases this development is backed by explicit national policies to strengthen the inclusion of peer support in service provision (Gillard et al 2015).

Peer support workers are defined in different ways, as 'peer providers', 'experiential experts', 'peer specialists', 'peer workers' and 'peer staff members'. In this chapter we refer to them as '*peer support workers*'. We define them as follows, with the above mentioned demarcation used by Repper and Carter (2011), as:

> Clients or former clients in mental health care who are trained and educated in formally recognized programs to transform their personal experience as a client into 'experiential knowledge' to help other clients, and who are formally employed as co-workers in professional teams.

There are claimed to be numerous benefits of the employment of peer support workers in different kind of mental health services (Crane and Lepicki 2016; Fisk et al 2000; Van Vugt et al 2012). Several studies show positive outcomes for clients. For example, peer support workers are expected to reduce the distance between service provision and clients, and to improve information sharing and understanding between professionals and service users (Agrawal et al 2016; Asad and Chreim 2016; Gillard et al 2015). Moreover, studies among clients indicate that the employment of peer support workers leads to less social isolation and a better quality of life, less hospitalisation and more independence and empowerment (Gates and Akabas 2007; Gillard et al 2015; Repper and Carter 2011). Finally, their involvement might facilitate system reform towards a more client-centred and recovery-oriented care (Agrawal et al 2016) as peer support workers can serve as a bridge between clients and the mental health system (Gillard et al 2015). Notwithstanding these positive effects, there are some studies that show no difference in outcomes between services with or without a peer support worker (Pitt et al 2013).

In sum, the use of experiential knowledge is gradually evolving into a generally valued and accepted way to achieve client centredness, and as a recognised part of treatment and care. However, its implementation is not without contestation, both because it is difficult to institutionalise a new occupation, especially in relation to existing professional fields, and it is difficult to formalise, use and 'insert' experiential knowledge, particularly in an era of expertise and evidence. How these dimensions of *control* and *content* – as key dimensions of professionalisation, seen as 'controlled content' (Noordegraaf 2007) – are played out during the professionalisation of peer support workers will be investigated in the following, based on empirical material from The Netherlands.

The rise and development of peer support workers in The Netherlands

Nowadays, the majority of the established and bigger mental health institutions in The Netherlands employs peer support workers. While precise numbers are unknown, the Dutch association for peer support workers *Vereniging voor Ervaringsdeskundigen* (VvED) reports an increase in the number of members and requests for advice from health care institutions regarding the employment of peer support workers. At the request of the Dutch Ministry of Health Care, in August 2019 the VvED began a research project to examine how many peer support workers are employed in mental health care settings (see www.vved.org).

Rough estimates speak of several hundred peer support workers who are employed in paid jobs in Dutch mental health care (Delespaul et al 2016). Many of them work in teams for 'Flexible Active Community Treatment', so-called *FACT teams*. This is a standardised treatment method, carried out by outreaching multidisciplinary teams, working for clients with chronic psychiatric illnesses. The FACT treatment model prescribes the employment of 1.2 (full-time) peer support workers per 200 clients (Van Vugt et al 2018). However, in practice most FACT teams do not comply with this standard (Boertien et al

2019). Teams usually have only one half-time employed peer support worker per 180–200 clients, and some teams do not have a peer support worker at all (Van Vugt et al 2018). Since there are around 300 FACT teams in The Netherlands (Van Vugt et al 2018) and as peer support workers also work in other settings, the aforementioned estimates seem plausible. Still, compared to regular professional groups in mental health care this is a very small number. For example, there are approximately 3,500 psychiatrists and 24,000 mental health nurses (Delespaul et al 2016) working among the 84,000 professionals in the mental health sector (Van Bakel et al 2013).

Next to FACT teams, peer support workers can also be found in settings for in-patient care (although they are much less frequently employed there) and in special services like peer recovery groups or so-called Recovery Colleges – centres that provide recovery support, training programmes and activities for people suffering from mental illness. More recently peer support workers have also emerged in other sectors and types of public services, such as youth care, debt assistance and poverty reduction teams.

Training and education

With the growing importance of peer support work, a wide range of training courses and educational programmes has developed, each focusing on a specific method or approach in peer support. First of all, there are short training courses, delivered by a variety of providers: client organisations, mental health institutions, recovery centres, and the like. Usually these training courses are facilitated by certified peer support workers, and bear titles such as 'Wellness Recovery Action Plan' (WRAP) or 'You heal yourself' (Boertien et al 2012). In addition, there are more formal professional education programmes such as 'Howie the Harp[TM]', originating from the United States, delivered by licensed providers in countries such as The Netherlands, usually by a mental health organisation. Based on a competency profile agreed at a national level, it prepares former clients in mental health care to work in a wide array of peer support roles, using the story of their own client experience. Contents range from theory on recovery to communication skills and from professional knowledge about mental illnesses to understanding team dynamics. Finally, over the years, long-term programmes have developed within the formal educational system, enabling students to acquire a formal degree as peer support workers. In The Netherlands there are several recognised institutions on both secondary level (so-called MBO) and higher educational level (HBO universities of applied science) that provide these programmes. The majority of peer support workers employed by mental health institutions are graduates from one of these formal graduate programmes.

Further development: the path to professionalisation?

Since peer support workers are increasingly visible in Dutch mental health care institutions, as they are given formal roles and as something is expected from them, they are expressing a strong desire for 'professionalisation'. This, at first sight, can be seen as a desire to establish formal recognition, to define a formal professional space – or 'jurisdiction' (Abbott 1988) – and to enact social closure in the labour market (Freidson 2001; Saks 2010). In that way, again at first sight, peer support work is gradually developing into an independent occupational and educational field (Boertien et al 2019). This formal desire for professionalisation manifests itself in a number of important ways.

First, together with mental health care institutions and their associations, colleges and educational institutes have developed initiatives to strengthen existing training *courses* for peer support workers and to provide uniformity as far as the *curricula* and *learning outcomes* are concerned. In 2013, moreover, a 'Professional Competency Profile' (Van Bakel et al 2013) for peer support workers was drafted, and subsequently transformed into a standard curriculum for peer support worker education. In 2017 and 2018 this was followed by more specific educational and didactic directives and programmes.

Second, support workers, represented by the VvED, are trying hard to achieve more formal registration. As one peer support worker has said: "The next step is to make clear that as a peer support worker, you think and act professionally" (Boer and Van der Pijl 2019: 16). This quote from a peer support worker refers to the efforts within the new occupational group to create a *professional register* for peer support workers. Such a register should make transparent who is entitled to call themself a professional peer support worker. In 2017 the VvED started a project to develop such a professional register, working together with a broad range of stakeholders, such as local and national client organisations, mental health and education institutions, the Dutch Ministry of Health Care and the branch association of health insurance companies. However, there are a lot of issues and dilemmas to be discussed and solved before realisation of this professional register becomes fact – for example, the risk that such a register will create (new) dividing lines within peer support workers as a group.

Third, there is increasing attention focused on support workers' payment. The lack of structural funding for their employment is a barrier to formal recognition of peer support workers as a profession. The Dutch health care financing system, legally anchored in (among other laws) the Health Insurance Law, does not recognise the profession of 'peer support worker'. As a consequence, their work is not 'billable'. As a result, many peer support workers, who are part of FACT teams, have had training in another health care profession to get around this financial barrier. In other cases, peer support workers are financed through 'overhead' or 'special budgets' made available by the institutions for which they work. The lack of structural funding basis is one of the reasons that the number of peer support workers in FACT teams has, so far, remained below the prescribed standard. At the policy level, this issue has received attention, for example in the policy agreement embodied in the General Agreement Mental Health Care 2019. This policy agreement, signed by the government, branch associations and professional associations, contains arrangements regarding funding experiments and future *structural financing* of peer support workers (Boertien et al 2019). As a consequence, the use of peer support workers should be billable by 2020.

In sum, the professionalisation of peer support workers materialises through several well-known mechanisms: the standardisation of the training; the protection and closure of the profession by way of formal registration, that is a professional register; and the establishment of structural funding. However, there is still a long road ahead, and in the meantime the position of peer support workers remains delicate and contested. All of this is part of the process of formal professionalisation at first sight. Nonetheless, when we dive deeper into the world of professionalising peer support workers, we have to focus on other developments. Apart from formal recognition and closure at an occupational level, other complicated issues and dilemmas are at stake, not least in the everyday realities of service delivery in well-organised surroundings (Asad and Chreim 2016; Gates and Akabas 2007; Gillard et al 2015). Peer support workers have to work together with other well established professionals, most specifically psychiatrists, psychologists and nurses, and they have to 'insert' their experiential knowledge in highly organised settings in which professional expertise and evidence are generally privileged. Apart from formal professionalisation, these realities of how 'controlled content' is enacted (Noordegraaf 2007) directly affect whether support workers are acting as new professionals and are recognised by their colleagues in established professions, or whether they are marginalised.

In the next two sections, one on 'control', the other on 'content', we shall highlight the actual team dynamics, by using empirical material from recent observational studies in Dutch mental health care. We initiated this study as there is little comparative research exploring real-life conditions that help or hinder peer support workers in taking up new roles (Gillard et al 2015). We shadowed multiple FACT teams which include peer support workers for several years. In particular, we observed their team meetings, and their deliberations and decision making process about issues regarding clients, to find out how experiential knowledge was used by peer support workers and professionals in these processes. Additionally, we conducted interviews with individual professionals and peer support workers, and we shadowed them during their face-to-face interactions with clients. This provided more specific insights into their opinions on peer support work and experiential knowledge, their interactions with clients, and the difference between professionals and peer support workers regarding these aspects of their work.

Peer support workers and mental health professionals: control

The roles of peer support workers are not undisputed and have been confronted with ambivalent responses from mental health professionals – psychiatrists, psychologists, nurses and therapists. Peer support workers may challenge the status and dominance of these traditional professionals, and they can affect professional powers and identities. In our study, set against insights coming from the few comparative studies that are available, we saw a number of control issues and dilemmas as set out in the following areas.

Lack of role clarity

There seems to be a lack of distinctiveness of peer support workers' roles, which is a widespread impediment to their incorporation in teams (Asad and Chreim 2016; Cabral et al 2014; Crane and Lepicki 2016; Ehrlich et al 2019; Fisk et al 2000; Gates and Akabas 2007; Gillard et al 2015; Hurley et al 2016; Moran et al 2013; Repper and Carter 2011). With reference to wider organisational role adoption literature, Gillard and colleagues (2015) point out that the lack of distinctiveness of a new role has been shown to mitigate successful role adoption. An extensive evaluation study into the use of peer support workers in mental health care teams in 18 mental health care institutions showed that such lack of role clarity is one of the most significant obstacles to the successful functioning of peer support workers in teams (Van Erp et al 2012). It raises questions such as: Are peer support workers mainly there to support the client, or should they primarily contribute to a more recovery-oriented mindset within the team? To what extent is the peer support worker expected to represent the client voice?

Despite the development of a job profile at national level, this lack of role clarity continues to be an issue for many mental health care practices. Moreover, this applies to both professionals and peer support workers themselves (Asad and Chreim 2016; Cabral et al 2014; Crane and Lepicki 2016; Gates and Akabas 2007; Gillard et al 2015; Repper and Carter 2011), as we found in our own study as well. Within the teams we observed, several professionals stated that they had no clear picture of the peer support worker's role or added value. A social worker in one of the teams expected the peer support worker to take up a more critical, activist role than she did, while the peer support worker herself stated in an interview that she 'did not want to be an activist'.

Dominant professional cultures

Alberta and colleagues (2012) identified both organisational and individual sets of challenges for peer support workers entering a professional work environment. Many professional staff members find it difficult to hand real control over service delivery process to peer support workers, as they work from an existing professional culture, mainly defined in terms of (academic) training and credentialing. Several authors (for example, Faulkner 2017; Hurley et al 2016; Vanderwalle et al 2016) state that the dominant paradigm in mental health care reflects the professional model, which is predicated on the existence of mental illness as having biomedical origins. As a result, peer support staff members have not always been taken seriously as full professionals. They may even be seen as 'junior staff' and be asked to perform futile tasks that are not linked to recovery (Alberta et al 2012; Moran et al 2013). Individual challenges include the inclination of peer support workers to act like their professionally trained co-workers, trying to fit in and gain professional recognition. In our study we saw comparable phenomena. For example, one of the peer support workers we observed and interviewed started her career in the team with a full-time contract as a peer support worker. As she was also trained as a social worker, and as payment was lower for peer support workers, she changed her contract (when the opportunity came) into a part-time position as a social worker and a part-time position as peer support worker. Only after that, she stated, did she feel completely recognised as a professional, both by herself and by the rest of the team.

Ambiguous identities

Several authors refer to the issue of ambiguous identities of peer support workers as an impediment to their acceptance as new professionals. Faulkner (2017) points out the risk of losing the characteristics of peer support workers if they take up roles as paid providers of services. She states that 'their roles can become removed from the experiential knowledge base that made them possible in the first place' (Faulkner 2017: 511). As such, peer support workers may risk co-optation in the professional group and culture in which they work (Alberta et al 2012), thus obscuring their peer identity. Fox (2016) raises the issue of 'double identity' – or rather, a blurring of boundaries between identities – as a service user and an academic lecturer on social work programmes. She states that it is unclear on what basis authority is founded in such cases – in lived experience or professional knowledge. As she puts it: 'My authority as an academic in the classroom is derived from my professional knowledge, yet it is the story of my lived experience that most inspires my students' (Fox 2016: 964). A wide range of literature on peer support workers in mental health shows that they often experience uncertainty about the boundaries between being a consumer and an employee or being a friend to fellow consumers and their service provider (Gates and Akabas 2007).

In our study, such ambiguity of, and in, identity was mentioned or shown by both professionals and peer support workers. To her regret, a mental health nurse in one of the teams observed that the peer support worker, since she accepted a part-time contract as a social worker, deployed her experiential knowledge less than before. Even more striking is the observation of two peer support workers who facilitated a peer group for clients. During the weekly meeting of the group, their attitude towards clients was ambiguous. They presented themselves to clients as fellow sufferers. They shared their own experiences – for instance, regarding 'quitting smoking' and 'feeling depressed' – as well as using the same language, and speaking in terms of 'us'. At the same time, however, they spoke more often than their clients, established rules ('there will be a break in 15 minutes, you can smoke then'), provided professional information, and sometimes adopted an advisory role.

Support workers' experiences and health professionals' expertise: content

When support workers bring experiential knowledge into decision making processes, there is no guaranteed outcome. Several substantive content issues emerging from both existing literature and our own study are at the root of this uncertain basis for the use of experiential knowledge, as documented in the following fields.

Experiential versus expert knowledge

Experiential knowledge, as a new form of knowledge that peer support workers introduce in the process of service delivery, turns out to be a problematic phenomenon. Faulkner (2017:509) defines it as 'knowledge based on the experience of service users and survivors'. Boevink (2017) describes it as a form of collective knowledge, based on stories of personal experience, about what it means to live with mental vulnerability and its consequences, and what helps or hinders the process of recovery. These concepts of knowledge differ strongly from prevailing knowledge concepts within established professions. Abbott (1988) asserts that professionalism is based on abstract knowledge, in which the higher the level of abstraction, the higher the level of professionalisation. Using this perspective, it comes as no surprise that tensions emerge between professionals on the one hand – who derive their status and discretionary powers from abstract, professional knowledge – and peer support workers on the other, who rely on a source of knowledge to which they assign a certain level of abstraction and value. Both experiential knowledge and its status in this context might be contested (also see, for instance, Baillergeau and Duyvendak 2016; Boevink 2017; Weerman 2016).

This issue is also present in the everyday practices of mental health care teams, as our own research showed. The professionals we interviewed recognised in general the value of the peer support worker's experiential knowledge, but at the same time there could be ambiguity about its specific or unique content. For example, a psychologist in one of the teams said: "I think in this team we all have experiential knowledge". Additionally, we observed that in their assessments and decision making professionals did not, or hardly ever, incorporate the knowledge provided by peer support workers. For example, during most team meetings peer support workers were seldom asked actively by the other team members to bring forward their opinion. Professionals appeared to value experiential knowledge predominantly when it concerned the *individual* relationship between peer support workers and clients. As one psychiatrist stated: "I am very positive about her role ... Peer support workers can discuss issues that patients don't discuss with me ..., but for us as professionals, it doesn't influence the way we look at patients". In short, we observed a *selective* use of experiential knowledge by professionals, notwithstanding their professed appreciation of its value.

Professional or organising responsibilities

One issue that turned out to be important in our own study is the nature and extent of formal professional responsibilities that are assigned to peer support workers. An example that we came across in our observation of the teams is bearing 'file responsibility'. For each client, there was always one professional (a nurse or social worker) who was the first contact person and who was responsible for keeping the files up-to-date. The file holder would also formulate the treatment plan, which had to be formally approved by the psychiatrist, together with the client. None of the peer support workers in our study bore this file responsibility. Such differences in responsibilities can have an impact on the status and position of peer support workers and can place them in an unwanted exceptional or inferior position in the team. Also, it might cause a certain envy among their professional co-workers, as a statement by a social worker in one of the teams illustrates:

> 'the moment a client is in crisis and derails, I am the one that has to pick her up with the ambulance, not the peer support worker. So I lose my equal relationship with the client. And he does have it ... It must be blissful to be able to work like that.'

Another type of responsibility concerns production targets. Perspectives on this matter were diverse in the teams that we studied. In a team where peer support workers had a fully-fledged production target, their relationship with professionals was fairly equal. A peer support worker in another team was completely exempt from such a production target, but played a marginal role in the team. A third team displayed a bit of both: the peer support worker also worked as a social worker and, while her role as peer support worker did not include a production target, her role as social worker did. She indicated that from that moment onwards she felt like she was taken more seriously. In short, our research shows that formal responsibilities also may determine the positioning of peer support workers.

This issue of formal professional responsibilities as a possible factor influencing the acceptance of peer support workers is hardly mentioned in literature on peer support work. Fox (2016) touches on the issue, citing an example from academic education. An academic teacher who also was a service user and used this experience in her teaching work was exempt from certain responsibilities associated with her professional role. The idea behind this was to enable her to focus her time on specific tasks associated with using her experiential knowledge, but as a consequence her authority and influence were diminished (Simons et al 2007). Crane and Lepicki (2016) studied differences in duties among peer support workers and case managers who fulfilled comparable support roles towards mental health clients and found that case managers had more formal duties, like performing administrative tasks. However, the focus in their study – and in many others – is more on tasks and duties than on formal responsibilities, although these aspects are interwoven.

Anxiety due to accountability

Finally, we came across an issue that is even less often mentioned in literature on peer support workers and their perspectives: the pressures of accountability for professionals and professional teams. Nowadays mental health institutions and teams are subject to a growing demand for transparency and accountability, as is the case in health care and other public services in general (Bovens et al 2016; Delespaul et al 2016; Noordegraaf 2011, 2015; Noordegraaf and Steijn 2013). This certainly has an impact on teams and their openness to client perspectives, as an example from our study illustrates. One of the nurses in a team we observed expressed his concerns about a client who often refused contact and gave verbal abuse. He wanted to take time to connect to her, but at the same time considered her an acute risk for other professionals. Recently a debt collector came to the client's door, but she denied him access and threatened him, while, as the nurse noticed, she kept an axe next to her front door. The nurse discussed the pressure for more coercive action towards the client with the team: "If we don't act, she will use that axe against the debt collector. Someone will be held accountable, and that will not be the debt collector."

Situations like this, combined with budget cuts, staff shortage – leading to extremely high caseloads – and a client population that is becoming more and more complex cause major pressures on teams and professionals in their day-to-day work, forcing them to be more coercive and directive towards clients than they would prefer. A quote from one of the interviewed psychiatrists underscores this point: "All this external pressure, police, others, demanding control … It doesn't go together with the idea of recovery." He expressed his disappointment at this situation, regretting the fact that the intentions to deliver more recovery-oriented care is kept down by the aforementioned accountability pressures, such that: "recovery then is a seed in barren soil".

Conclusion

When we take the control and content issues that we observed in day-to-day service delivery in mental health teams into account, we can shed more refined light on the actual and potential professionalisation process of peer support workers. In the first part of this chapter, we showed that there is much stress on traditional notions of professionalism when the formal process of strengthening peer support work is analysed. This implies that the process focuses on strengthening occupational control, by establishing schooling, certification, registration and standardisation. On the basis of our empirical observational research, however, we later showed that *organisational* conditions count, much more than *occupational* conditions. Peer support workers face a lack of role clarity, strong professional cultures, ambiguous identities, a lack of status, unclear responsibilities and accountability pressures.

This means that not so much *more* but *other* efforts can be made by this new occupational group to position themselves in well-organised service surroundings. It also means that organisations and professional teams should pay explicit attention to the organisational role and responsibilities of peer support workers when they are employed to improve client-centred service delivery. When we focus on the everyday realities of how peer support workers work in teams, we have to be sensitive to how the usage of experiential knowledge is *organised*, in relation to contexts that do not automatically accept peer support workers, both in terms of who they are and what they know, first and foremost as perceived by others. Their roles, routines and identities are not automatically accepted, and their status, responsibilities and effectiveness are not automatically clear. This is exacerbated as they work in relation to clients, who have 'client autonomy'; together with other rather more autonomous health professionals who are part of existing professional fields; and in broader organisational surroundings full of autonomous optimisation processes.

This underscores the importance of new images of professionalism, which go beyond traditional images of autonomous professionals based on neo-Weberian concepts of social closure who know how to act professionally. It also calls for new competencies or capabilities, most specifically so-called *organising* capabilities (Noordegraaf 2015; Noordegraaf et al 2014). The interweaving of new forms of knowledge – such as experiential knowledge – in ongoing service processes in well-organised surroundings does not happen spontaneously, but has to be consciously *organised*. Both professionals and peer support workers should be involved in this process. For professionals it implies a broadening of their professional authority (Noordegraaf 2007). Being capable to organise the use or synthesis of different kinds of knowledge could be part of their professionalism, and securing connections to stakeholders – in this case specifically clients and their peer support worker representatives – could be taken up more fully as an active responsibility for professionals. For peer support workers this means that their experiential knowledge *per se* is not really meaningful. How their knowledge and experiences are woven into the fabric of organised service delivery by teams and for multiple clients makes them meaningful. Peer support workers have to work on who they are and what they know. They have to make sure that both clients and colleagues see their added value, and that they are well-positioned and taken seriously. In short, peer support workers have to more professionally organise their work in order to work in professional organisations.

References

Abbott, A. (1988) *The System of Professions. An Essay on the Division of Expert Labor*, Chicago, IL: University of Chicago Press.

Agrawal, S., Capponi, P., Lopez, J., Kidd, S., Ringsted, C., Wiljer, D. and Soklaridis, S. (2016) 'From surviving to advising: A novel course pairing mental health and addiction service users as advisors to senior psychiatry residents', *Academic Psychiatry* 40: 475–80.

Alberta, A.J., Ploski, R.R. and Carlson, S.L. (2012) 'Addressing challenges to providing peer-based recovery support', *Journal of Behavioral Health Services and Research* 39(4): 481–91.

Asad, S. and Chreim, S. (2016) 'Peer support providers' role experiences on interprofessional mental health care teams: A qualitative study', *Community Mental Health Journal* 52: 767–74.

Baillergeau, E. and Duyvendak, J.W. (2016) 'Experiential knowledge as a resource for coping with uncertainty: Evidence and examples from the Netherlands', *Health, Risk and Society* 18(7–8): 407–26.

Baklien, B. and Bongaardt, R. (2014) 'The quest for choice and the need for relational care in mental health work', *Medicine, Health Care and Philosophy* 17: 625–32.

Boer, M. and Van der Pijl, K. (2019) 'Beroepsregistratie ervaringsdeskundigen', *Participatie en Herstel* 28(1): 15–24.

Boertien, D., Van Bakel, M. and Van Weeghel, J. (2012) 'Wellness recovery action plan in Nederland – Een herstelmethode bij psychische ontwrichting', *Maandblad Geestelijke Volksgezondheid* 67(5): 276–83.

Boertien, D., Wadman, H. and Hulshof, E. (2019) 'Reflecties op de inhoudelijke ontwikkeling van ervaringsdeskundigheid', *Participatie en Herstel* 28(1): 3–14.

Boevink, W. (2017) *Planting a Tree. On Recovery, Empowerment and Experiential Expertise*, Utrecht: Trimbos Netherlands Institute of Mental Health and Addiction.

Bovens, M., Goodin, R.E. and Schillemans, T. (eds) (2016) *The Oxford Handbook of Public Accountability*, Oxford: Oxford University Press.

Cabral, L., Strother, H., Muhr, K., Sefton, L. and Savageau, J. (2014) 'Clarifying the role of the mental health peer specialist in Massachusetts, USA: Insights from peer specialist, supervisors and clients', *Health and Social Care in the Community* 22(1): 104–12.

Crane, D.A. and Lepicki, T. (2016) 'Unique and common elements of the role of peer support in the context of traditional mental health services', *Psychiatric Rehabilitation Journal* 39(30): 282–8.

Delespaul, P., Milo, M., Schalken, F., Boevink, W. and Van Os, J. (2016) *Goede GGZ! Nieuwe concepten, aangepaste taal en betere organisatie*, Leusden: Diagnose Uitgevers.

Dixon, L., Krauss, N. and Lehman, A. (1994) 'Consumers as service providers: The promise and challenge', *Community Mental Health Journal* 30(6): 615–25.

Ehrlich, C., Slattery, M., Vilic, G., Chester, P. and Crompton, D.D. (2019) 'What happens when peer support workers are introduced as members of community-based clinical mental health service delivery teams: a qualitative study', *Journal of Interprofessional Care*, https://doi.org/10.1080/13561820.2019.1612334

Faulkner, A. (2017) 'Survivor research and mad studies: The role and value of experiential knowledge in mental health research', *Disability and Society* 32(4): 500–20.

Fisk, D., Rowe, M., Brooks, R. and Gildersleeve, D. (2000) 'Integrating consumer staff members into a homeless outreach project: Critical issues and strategies', *Psychiatric Rehabilitation Journal* 23(3): 244.

Fox, J. (2016) 'Being a service user and a social work academic: Balancing expert identities', *Social Work Education* 35(8): 960–69.

Freidson, E. (2001) *Professionalism: The Third Logic*, Cambridge: Polity Press.

Gates, L.B. and Akabas, S.H. (2007) 'Developing strategies to integrate peer providers into the staff of mental health agencies', *Administration and Policy in Mental Health* 34: 293–306.

Gillard, S., Holley, J. Gibson, S., Larsen, J., Lucock, M., Oborn, E., Rinaldi, M. and Stamou, E. (2015) 'Introducing new peer worker roles into mental health services in England: Comparative case study research across a range of organizational contexts', *Administration and Policy in Mental Health* 42: 682–94.

Hunt, M.G. and Resnick, S.G. (2015) 'Two birds, one stone: Unintended consequences and a potential solution for problems with recovery in mental health', *Psychiatric Services* 66(11): 1235–37.

Hurley, J., Cashin, A., Mills, J., Hutchinson, M. and Graham, I. (2016) 'A critical discussion of peer workers: Implications for the mental health nursing workforce', *Journal of Psychiatric and Mental Health Nursing* 23: 129–35.

McMurray, R. (2010) 'The struggle to professionalize: An ethnographic account of the occupational position of Advanced Nurse Practitioners', *Human Relations* 64(6): 801–22.

Moran, G.S., Russinova, Z., Gidugu, V. and Gagne, C. (2013) 'Challenges experienced by paid peer providers in mental health recovery: A qualitative study', *Community Mental Health Journal* 49: 281–91.

Mowbray, C.T., Moxley, D.P., Thrasher, D.S.W., Bybee, D., McCrohan, N., Harris, S. and Clover, G. (1996) 'Consumers as community support providers: Issues created by role innovation', *Community Mental Health Journal* 32(1): 47–67.

Noordegraaf, M. (2007) 'From "pure" to "hybrid" professionalism. Present-day professionalism in ambiguous public domains', *Administration and Society* 39(6): 761–85.

Noordegraaf, M. (2011) 'Risky business. How professionals and professionals fields (must) deal with organizational issues', *Organization Studies* 32: 1349–71.

Noordegraaf, M. (2015) 'Hybrid professionalism and beyond. (New) forms of public professionalism in changing organizational and societal contexts', *Journal of Professions and Organization* 2(2): 187–206.

Noordegraaf, M. and Steijn, B. (eds) (2013) *Professionals under Pressure. The Reconfiguration of Professional Work in Changing Public Services*, Amsterdam: Amsterdam University Press.

Noordegraaf, M., Van der Steen, M. and Twist, M.J.W. (2014) 'Fragmented or connective professionalism? Strategies for professionalizing the work of strategists and other (organizational) professionals', *Public Administration* 92(1): 21–38.

Pitt, V., Lowe, D., Prictor, M., Hetrick, S.E., Ryan, R. and Berends, L. (2013) 'Consumer-providers of care for adult clients of statutory mental health services (Review)', *Cochrane Database of Systematic Reviews* 3: 1–104.

Repper, J. and Carter, T. (2011) 'A review of the literature on peer support in mental health services', *Journal of Mental Health* 20(4): 392–411.

Saks, M. (2010) 'Analyzing the professions: The case for the neo-Weberian approach', *Comparative Sociology* 9: 887–915.

Simons, L., Tee, S., Lathlean, J., Burgess, A., Herbert, L. and Gibson, C. (2007) 'A socially inclusive approach to user participation in higher education', *Journal of Advanced Nursing* 58: 246–55.

Tholen, G. (2017) 'The changing opportunities of professionalization for graduate occupations', *Comparative Sociology* 16: 613–33.

Van Bakel, M., Van Rooijen, S., Boertien, D., Kamoschinski, J., Liefhebber, S. and Kluft, M. (2013) *Ervaringsdeskundigheid Beroepscompetentieprofiel*, Utrecht: GGz Nederland, Trimbos Netherlands Institute of Mental Health and Addiction, HEE! and Kenniscentrum Phrenos.

Van Erp, N., Rijkaart, A.M., Boertien, D., Van Bakel, M. and Van Rooijen, S. (2012) *Vernieuwende inzet van ervaringsdeskundigheid. Evaluatieonderzoek in 18 ggz-instellingen*, Utrecht: Trimbos Netherlands Institute of Mental Health and Addiction.

Van Vugt, M., Kroon, H., Delespaul, P.A.E.G. and Mulder, C.L. (2012) 'Consumer-providers in Assertive Community Treatment programs: associations with client outcomes', *Psychiatric Services* 63(5): 477–81.

Van Vugt, M., Mulder, N., Bahler, M., Delespaul, P., Westen, K. and Kroon, H. (2018) 'Modelgetrouwheid van flexible assertive community treatment (FACT) teams: resultaten van vijf jaar auditeren', *Tijdschrift voor Psychiatrie* 60(7): 441–8.

Vanderwalle, J., Debyser, B., Beeckman, D., Vandecasteele, T., Van Hecke, A. and Verhaeghe, S. (2016) 'Peer workers' perceptions and experiences of barriers to implementation of peer worker roles in mental health services: A literature review', *International Journal of Nursing Studies* 60: 234–50.

Weerman, A. (2016) *Ervaringsdeskundige zorg- en dienstverleners. Stigma, verslaving en existentiële transformatie*, Utrecht: Eburon.

NINE

Complementary and alternative medicine as an invisible health support workforce

Joana Almeida and Nelson Barros

Introduction

Complementary and alternative medicine (CAM) is a complex phenomenon and difficult to define. According to the World Health Organization (WHO) (2013:15), 'the terms "complementary medicine" or "alternative medicine" refer to a broad set of health care practices that are not part of that country's own tradition or conventional medicine and are not fully integrated into the dominant healthcare system'. The WHO (2013:7) also states that CAM 'is an important and often underestimated part of healthcare … found in almost every country in the world and the demand for its services is increasing'. In this chapter CAM is analysed in terms of its links to health support work.

From the point of view of the sociology of professions, the term CAM includes, at one end of the spectrum, statutorily regulated and professionalised therapies such as osteopathy and chiropractic in the UK which have achieved exclusionary social closure in neo-Weberian terms (Saks 2008). Further along the line are acupuncture and homeopathy, which, although not statutorily regulated, have their own voluntary self-regulatory bodies, such as the British Acupuncture Council and the British Homeopathic Association. At the other end of the spectrum are those CAM therapies less disposed to professionalisation, usually not regulated by the state, lacking consistent educational standards and with a strong emphasis on self-help, such as reiki and yoga (Saks 2008). To add to this, the status of CAM varies across countries. Traditional acupuncturists, for example, are statutorily regulated in Canada (Ijaz et al 2016), but not in the UK, despite being governed by limited local by-laws (Saks 1995).

A similar conceptual ambiguity exists with respect to health support workers more generally. The latter include not only those unqualified workers who assist professionally qualified health care workers in the delivery of care, but also those who are providers of care themselves – such as the case of CAM practitioners working in the private sector directly paid by service users. As stated by Manthorpe and Martineau (2008:4–5):

> ... tasks performed [by support workers] will depend on the specific type of support worker under consideration and the wishes and needs of the person they support, and may range from personal care, healthcare, community participation, assistance in rehabilitation and advocacy.

The diversity of regulatory status of CAM practices and practitioners across countries, and of support worker roles, therefore, makes it difficult to generalise. Thus, to depict the status and position of CAM practitioners as straight forwardly being support workers in health care should be undertaken with caution.

There is a gap in sociological research on the similarities in status and market position of CAM practitioners and health support workers when compared to other professionally qualified health care professions. The literature predominantly focuses on health care assistants, personal assistants, social work assistants, home care support workers, rehabilitation workers, mental health support workers, and community support workers (Manthorpe and Martineau 2008). This chapter helps to fill this vacuum by critically exploring the extent to which CAM practitioners have formed part of this undervalued and invisible health support workforce. In so doing, commonalities between CAM practitioners and health support workers will be highlighted, focusing on the social closure theory of the professions, and on the interlinked societies of Brazil and Portugal as illustrative contexts.

Health support work and complementary and alternative medicine

Increasing numbers of people have been employed as 'support workers' in public and private health care in Western societies. They have been termed the 'frontline staff' (Cavendish 2013), providing a substantial amount of hands-on care. According to the Health Education England (HEE) review of care staff and registered nurses, health support workers make up well over 1 million of the total British national health system workforce, and 60 per cent of health support workers are providers of care (HEE 2015). Yet they remain invisible and a minority group when it comes to the distribution of the national training budget. The growth of such a workforce has arisen from several factors, including the increasing ageing population living with chronic conditions, and the need to provide personal care to them (Sarre et al 2018). As stated by the HEE (2015:14): 'the increasing level of vulnerability associated with complex needs and an ageing population requires a particular focus on compassionate care'.

Recent neo-liberal policies have also found cheaper forms of health care labour through the enhancement of status, income and power, substitution, the delegation of tasks, and innovation (Saks 2008). This has led to an increase of health support workers, as well as a growing concern with their educational and training standards and the conduct of these workers (Cavendish 2013). In their qualitative study of experiences of health care support workers in three English hospitals, Sarre and colleagues (2018) found discontentment with training, shadowing and mentoring provision, development opportunities, and the lack of enthusiasm of ward managers for support worker training. Inadequate infrastructures, frequently poorly funded training, low wages, uncertain terms and conditions of work, unclear job descriptions, blurred professional boundaries, and lack of regulation were also pointed out by Manthorpe and Martineau (2008) in their review of support workers.

Although very little still is known about the role, motivations and employment conditions of health support workers, they are often perceived as a low qualified group, without statutory regulation, accreditation, and mandatory registers, including a limited number of occupations with voluntary registers. Manthorpe and Martineau (2008) claim that support work is an ill-defined concept, with problems of role definition and role overlap and hybridity with other professionals. Even so, they identify three main characteristics present in support work occupations: "first, fostering independence among people being 'supported'; secondly, such workers are generally without professional accreditation; thirdly, they frequently engage in both social care and healthcare tasks, or wider tasks" (Manthorpe and Martineau 2008:4). These authors also state that being approachable, practical and emotionally supportive, and able to extend their social contact with service users, was one advantage of support workers in relation to professionally qualified health care staff. Moreover, the service user's general satisfaction with the absence of professional characteristics of support workers raises questions about the value of stricter future regulation and professionalisation of these workers.

Health support work can also be defined as involving 'marginalised' and, most importantly, 'marginal' work. This, on the one hand, includes professions with a subordinated status (like nurses and physiotherapists) and/or limited power and income (like opticians, dentists or pharmacists), as compared to medical doctors. More crucially in this context, this category encompasses groups which operate outside state support and are excluded from the mainstream health care workforce (Saks 2015). This applies to most CAM practitioners in countries like the UK, Australia and the United States, among others. Variations in support worker roles and training levels across health care settings have not contributed towards the regulation of such work.

Another important aspect of support work is its increased presence in compassionate, preventative and palliative care. As stated by Manthorpe and Martineau (2008:9): 'the goal of intermediate care [in which support work has developed] is the prevention of unnecessary hospital stays and the avoidance of premature or needless admissions'. In other words, the support worker is the intermediary between the service user and qualified professionals. The UK NHS certainly includes such intermediary CAM practitioners within the category of 'clinical support workers' (NHS Health Careers 2019). The NHS differentiates here between 'supporting registered practitioners', such as health assistants and occupational therapists, 'professional clinical support', such as nutritionists and CAM practitioners, 'specialist clinical support' and a range of other roles which do not need a particular qualifications, such as dental support workers (NHS Health Careers 2019). From a neo-Weberian perspective, the NHS recognition of CAM support workers has resulted from ongoing jurisdictional and legitimacy battles between CAM practitioners, other professionally qualified health care professions such as the medical profession, and the state. It is to this struggle that we now turn.

Complementary and alternative medicine support workers and social closure

According to a neo-Weberian approach, interprofessional relationships are conflictual in relation to power and interests. Professionalised and professionalising groups engage in a struggle to gain occupational closure through jurisdictional battles (Saks 1996). These jurisdictional battles are translated into tacit strategies which are used to maintain, gain or restrict jurisdictional control. Witz (1992) identifies inclusionary usurpation and dual closure strategies, which are primary strategies employed by subordinate occupational groups such as CAM support workers in response to their outsider status.

She also identifies exclusionary and demarcationary strategies, which are typically pursued by dominant occupational groups such as the medical profession that strive to maintain their monopolistic control over knowledge systems in order to restrict access to rewards and privileges by outsider groups.

In their study of British homeopathy, Cant and Sharma (1996) demonstrated the engagement in strategies of inclusion and dual closure by non-medically qualified homeopaths. As the authors stated, these practitioners, after working for years without a structured knowledge system, started to engage in accreditation processes – through the establishment of standards of training and practice taught in recognised courses in accredited colleges. Simultaneously they dropped their more controversial teaching in order to acquire higher recognition by medical orthodoxy, the state and the public. They have also engaged in a dual closure process, by demarcating and protecting their expertise from biomedicine, but also from potentially dangerous, dubious and non-qualified homeopathic practitioners. This resembles the status of health support workers in general, who conventionally are understood to not have professional accreditation, yet carry out generic and diverse tasks, with blurred boundaries between health and social care (Manthorpe and Martineau 2008), despite increased scrutiny of, and policy attention on, their role and training (Sarre et al 2018).

Nowadays homeopathy has seen a decline in the UK. The Science and Technology Committee report by the House of Commons (2010) on homeopathy stated that homeopathic products perform like a placebo, and NHS England and NHS Clinical Commissioners (2017) concluded that homeopathic remedies should be de-prescribed in primary health care, following a review of the use of homeopathy in the NHS. The same has happened to acupuncture, which is no longer recommended by the National Institute for Health and Care Excellence (NICE) for managing low back pain, with or without sciatica, due to evidence showing that this therapy is no more effective than sham treatment (NICE 2016). The rhetoric of CAM's lack of scientific evidence has been one of the most effective ways for the medical profession to achieve occupational exclusion and demarcation, as a dominant professional group (Kelner et al 2004). Furthermore, the scientific criteria of exclusion by biomedicine are embedded in formal organisations of civil society, such as universities, hospitals, laboratories and clinics. Medical students engage in a long period of schooling and training based on a scientific paradigm and a body of theory. Work in hospitals and clinics is similarly 'aligned with science' (Welsh et al 2004:219). As Halpern (1990) notes, biomedicine holds a higher degree of influence over the organisation of medical workplaces as well as sufficient authority to shape the division of labour in health care.

Important to this discussion too is the concept of strategy. Saks (1995) suggested a shift, by the mid-1970s, in the medical reception of acupuncture in Britain in the wake of increasing user demand from the rejection of CAM to its increasing medical incorporation and to the limitation of CAM practitioners only to certain health conditions. Biomedicine legitimised this therapy through neurophysiological explanations about the way it works, and its delimitation to the management of pain. At the time of writing, on the webpage of the British Medical Acupuncture Society (BMAS), there is reference to 'Western medical acupuncture', which is defined as an adaptation of Chinese acupuncture by using current, up-to-date knowledge of anatomy, physiology and pathology, and the principles of evidence-based medicine (BMAS 2019).

This alignment of the medical profession with CAM was anticipated five decades ago by Levy (1966), who had already stated that biomedical resistance to osteopaths and chiropractors would decrease if the medical profession limited the care of those practitioners to back pain caused by a structural defect of the spinal column. For Levy, osteopaths and chiropractors would follow the same trend as other health support workers who were circumscribed to specific tasks or areas of health. This 'tacit acknowledgment' (Wiese et al 2010) of CAM is a way of maintaining its complementary and subordinate status, by retaining medical power to decide when a patient should be referred to an alternative practitioner and employing a 'delegation' strategy. Nowadays, osteopaths and chiropractors are the only CAM practitioners statutorily regulated in the UK, yet they remain marginalised, usually practising privately and/or employed by direct payment by users, like many health support workers. As suggested by Saks (1996), CAM practitioners have moved to becoming 'deviant insiders' from 'unorthodox outsiders', as they have started integrating into mainstream health care, albeit under biomedical sovereignty.

The issue of the subjugated segregation of CAM support workers is important, as it accounts for the 'distinction between the adoption of therapies on the one hand, and recognition of therapists on the other' (Siahpush 1999:172). Nevertheless, in one way or another, CAM practices and practitioners remain marginalised and/or subordinated to the medical profession and its biomedical logic in the UK and many other Western societies (Polich et al 2010). The literature presented here therefore highlights the way in which CAM practitioners have formed part of a marginalised and invisible health support workforce – even if its positioning is not always a straight forward fit. By way of further illustration, we now discuss the standing of CAM practices and practitioners in the interrelated societies of Brazil and Portugal.

Complementary and alternative medicine in Brazil

Brazil is a South American country and a federative republic composed of 26 states and one federal district. Each state is divided into administrative regions, called municipalities. There are 5,570 municipalities in the country. The Brazilian constitution established the Unified Health System (Systemic Único de Saúde in Portuguese, known as the SUS) in 1988, after two decades of military dictatorship in the country. The SUS was founded based on three main principles: integrality, equity, and universality. It is a decentralised health system, with states and municipalities having full autonomy and control over health care management and providing comprehensive and free health care to the whole population.

A main aspect of the SUS is its emphasis on prevention and rehabilitation. In 1994 the Family Health Programme (Programa Saúde da Família, later reworded Estratégia Saúde da Família (ESF) or Family Health Strategy) was created to improve primary health care. This strategy was implemented through multi-professional teams, originally consisting of a general practitioner, a nurse, an auxiliary nurse, and 4–6 community health workers, all working in primary health care units (Durão and Menezes 2016; Harris and Haines 2010). An extended version of these multi-professional teams in some municipalities might also include a surgeon dentist, and a dentist assistant and/or a dentist technician. The Family Health Strategy is an attempt to revive a holistic health and social care approach, where community-based primary health care is fostered mainly through the employment of community health workers. Community health workers had a crucial role in the inception of the ESF, due to their strong links with the community. However, the status of these workers has recently changed through Directive 2.436/2017 (Brazilian Ministry of Health 2017c), where it is stated that their inclusion within ESF teams becomes optional.

It was also during the 1980s and 1990s that political interest in the regulation of specific CAM practices started in the country. Many governmental meetings and national health conferences were held with the aim of recommending the incorporation of specific CAM practices into primary health care. As a result, in 2003 under the government of ex-President Lula da Silva, a working group comprising representatives of national associations of herbal medicine, homeopathy, acupuncture and anthroposophical medicine, and the Ministry of Health was set up, with the aim of discussing and creating a national policy for CAM practices – where 'integrative and complementary practices' is the country-specific nomenclature for CAM.

In 2006 the National Policy for Integrative and Complementary Practices (PNPIC) was approved within the SUS. This policy regulated five integrative and complementary practices – traditional Chinese medicine/acupuncture, homeopathy, herbal medicine, anthroposophical medicine and thermalism/crenotherapy – given the increasing use and demand for these therapies by service users, as well as the important services they could provide in areas such as health promotion, prevention and rehabilitation within the SUS (Almeida et al 2018a). In 2011 these CAM practices were rolled out by the Health Academy Programme launched by the Ministry of Health through Directive 719/2011, as a way of promoting health care and healthy lifestyles (Brazilian Ministry of Health 2011). In 2017 14 other CAM therapies were added to the list by the Ministry of Health (Directive 849/2017), as a result of a governmental review of primary care teams, based on the Programme for Improving Primary Care Access and Quality (PMAQ). The review concluded that different CAM practices had been used by 30,000 primary health care teams across the country and the following CAM therapies were added to the SUS: art therapy, Ayurvedic medicine, biodance, chiropractic, circular dance, integrative community therapy, meditation, music therapy, naturopathy, osteopathy, reflexotherapy, reiki, shantala and yoga (Brazilian Ministry of Health 2017a). In March 2018 this list was further extended, when ten new integrative and complementary practices were added (Directive 702/2018), including hypnotherapy, aromatherapy and bioenergy (Brazilian Ministry of Health 2018).

At present, a total of 29 integrative and complementary practices have entered the SUS. Although mainly available within primary health care, some of them have also been offered in the secondary and tertiary health care sectors. CAM practices have therefore been available in 54 per cent of the municipalities across the 26 states and federal districts – 78 per cent in primary care, 18 per cent in specialised care and 4 per cent in hospital care (Brazilian Ministry of Health 2017b). According to the Brazilian Ministry of Health, since the implementation of the PNPIC in the SUS in 2006, the use of CAM practices has significantly increased. In 2016 more than 2 million CAM consultations took place in all the country's primary care units, including 770,000 in traditional Chinese medicine and acupuncture, 85,000 in phytotherapy, 13,000 in homeopathy and 923,000 in other practices not yet considered by Brazilian CAM legislation (Brazilian Ministry of Health 2019). Such practices can best be regarded as outside the realm of health support work as, although they are providing popular complementary, if marginal, services, they are typically delivered by professional staff within the SUS.

The practice of *tai chi chuan* by primary health care professionals also grew between 2017 and 2018, which, together with yoga, saw an increase of 46 per cent (Brazilian Ministry of Health 2017b). Similarly, and during the same time span, auriculotherapy consultations more than doubled from 157,000 to 355,000, greater than a 126 per cent increase (Brazilian Ministry of Health 2017b, 2017c). Like *tai chi*, auriculotherapy is not included in the 29 CAM practices regulated within the SUS, as it is seen as part of traditional Chinese medicine. Nonetheless, the National Committee for Complementary and Integrative Health Practices (Comissão Nacional de Práticas Integrativas e Complementares em Saúde, known as CNPICS), part of the Ministry of Health, together with the Federal University of Sta Catarina, in the state of Florianopolis, has launched auriculotherapy courses for primary health care professionals since 2016. These have been offered in 19 settings across 12 states, and in 2018 more than 4,000 health care professionals have enrolled in it (CNPICS 2018; Tesser et al 2019), including community health workers.

An example which more forcefully illustrates the marginality of CAM outside the SUS is *lian gong*, a collective body practice with origins in traditional Chinese medicine. In the 20 municipalities which make up the metropolitan region of Campinas (with 3.5 million inhabitants), it is the most prevalent CAM practice, being present in 98 out of 117 primary health care centres offering CAM out of a total of 236 primary care centres in the region (Barros et al 2016). *Lian gong* is also not included among the 29 CAM practices regulated within the SUS. Oliveira (2018) shows that most of the *lian gong* practitioners in the metropolitan region of Campinas are female community health workers, whose integration within the multi-professional teams is perceived as precarious. The community health workers interviewed explained such precarity through conflicts between CAM practices and other 'priority' tasks, the accumulation of roles, lack of practitioners with expertise in CAM, lack of institutional support, and limited physical space to practice *lian gong*. Barros and colleagues (2018) have also come to the same conclusions in their mapping of the CAM offer across primary health care centres. They show that primary care service coordinators are aware of the low visibility and recognition of CAM practices and practitioners by other ESF team members who support more orthodox health care – reflecting one of the characteristics of health support work.

The Brazilian state thus has regulated a fair amount of CAM practices recently, but only those that can be practised within the SUS. Alongside this expansion of CAM within the SUS, there has been an increase in the numbers of traditional non-medically qualified CAM practitioners, who are often self-regulated and have provided their services outside the SUS in the private health care market. According to the International Society of Therapists (Sociedade Internacional de Terapia, known as SINTE), there are around 150,000 such holistic therapists who more strongly bear the mark of health support workers in the sense adopted in this volume, including acupuncturists, floral therapists, herbal therapists, aestheticians, body therapists, chiropractors, orthomolecular therapists and reiki therapists (SINTE 2016). They are not statutorily regulated, and have acquired diverse training and qualifications, usually provided by their associations and organisations. The number of these voluntary associations offering safety and ethical standards and legal advice to protect the practice of a variety of CAM therapies has increased since the 1990s (Almeida et al 2018a). Examples are the SINTE and its trade union, founded in 1992. This Society voluntarily regulates 'holistic therapists' and claims to be the only national association representing such practitioners in the country (SINTE 2016). The SINTE issues the Credentialed Holistic Therapist Licence and Technical Norms for the exercise of holistic therapy. Nevertheless, the Brazilian Association of Holistic Therapists, created in 2007, also aims to regulate holistic therapists and issues a Certificate of Technical Responsibility to its affiliates.

In summary, with reference to the practice of CAM in Brazil, 29 CAM therapies have been statutorily regulated to be used by primary health care professionals, including medical doctors, nurses, dentists, and community health workers. However, the use of these therapies within the ESF's multi-professional teams has been neglected and marginalised, in favour of biomedical practices and modes of organisation. CAM therapists, who work outside the SUS and more strongly take on the characteristic of health support workers, have also been marginal and invisible to the public health care system. Crucially, they lack state regulation in terms of social closure – thus mirroring the position of health support workers more generally. The chapter now turns to examine the extent to which CAM can be regarded as a type of health support work in Portugal.

Complementary and alternative medicine in Portugal

Portugal is a Southern European country and has been a semi-presidential parliamentary republic since 1974. The country has a national health care service (Serviço Nacional de Saúde, known as the SNS), financed mainly through taxation and established in 1979. Act 56/79 guarantees the right to health protection and free access to health care to everyone, irrespective of their socioeconomic status. The Central Administration of the Health System (ACSS) manages the human and financial resources of the Ministry of Health and the SNS. The A3ES (Agência de Avaliação e Acreditação do Ensino Superior) is an independent public agency founded in 2007 by Decree 369/2007, which is responsible for the evaluation and accreditation of higher education institutions and respective degrees in the country. The Portuguese Medical Council is the professional body that oversees medical practice in the country.

CAM regulation in Portugal started in the late 1990s, with the publication in 1999 of a CAM report written by a working group formed with representatives of the Ministry of Health, the Medical and Pharmaceutical Councils, the General Directorate of Higher Education (Direcção-Geral do Ensino Superior) and the Department of Human Resources for Health (Departamento de Recursos Humanos da Saúde), thus excluding any CAM representatives. The report addressed the status of CAM in the country and worldwide, advising on the statutory regulation of CAM practices and practitioners. This report led to much controversy between the state, the medical profession, and CAM representatives, as well as to political action which resulted in the publication of Act 45/2003 that regulates six CAM professions: acupuncture, homeopathy, osteopathy, chiropractic, naturopathy and phytotherapy (Almeida and Gabe 2016). Due to various factors, including short periods of national political instability and austerity, as well as disagreements among members of the working group set up to advise on CAM regulation, this legislation was regulated only ten years later by Act 71/2013. Act 71/2013 regulates those same six professions, and traditional Chinese medicine, which was added to the list. 'Non-conventional therapeutics' is the country-specific nomenclature for CAM.

Act 71/2013 establishes that the exercise of the seven professions is permitted only to those registered with the ACSS and therefore holding a professional licence accredited and issued by the ACSS itself. In other words, only those practitioners holding such a licence can use the title of 'specialist' in acupuncture, homeopathy, osteopathy, chiropractic, naturopathy, phytotherapy and traditional Chinese medicine. Thus, as stated by Act 71/2013, in order to become a CAM professional accredited by the state, a higher education degree at polytechnic level is required, of which length and content are to be jointly determined and published by the Ministry of Health and the Ministry of Higher Education. Act 71/2013 also states that those CAM practitioners who were already working in one of the seven CAMs by the time of Act 71/2013 came into force, would have their qualification and training subject to scrutiny in order to evaluate their standards and licence to practise CAM in the health market (Assembleia da República Portuguesa 2013). Similarly, schools which, at the time of the Act, had been providing training and qualification in one of the seven CAM therapies, would have a 5-year transitional period to adapt to the new legislation and thus to upgrade to higher education institutions. This is still to happen. In fact, in 2019 the President of the Republic vetoed a bill on the formation of the School of Non-Conventional Therapeutics in Coimbra, by stating that 'the competent professional Councils have not approved the teaching of non-conventional medicines [CAM], as there is no scientific evidence of their effectiveness; furthermore, in countries where [CAM] teaching had been liberated, they have backtracked' (Presidência da República 2019). It is unclear to which countries President Sousa is making reference, but they could include the case of the UK, where recent government reports have discouraged the practice of homeopathy (House of Commons 2010) and acupuncture in primary health care (NICE 2016).

In 2014 the government published the requirements for obtaining a professional licence to practice CAM therapies in the country, through Directives 182-A/2014 and 182-B/2014. The legal document states that a €60 fee should be paid to register with the A3ES and obtain a licence to practise. In 2014 the competences and rules for a CAM Consultative Council, as well as the Council's members, were set out by Directives 25/2014 and 12337/2014 respectively. Once again this Council witnessed much internal turbulence not only between CAM representatives and representatives of the medical profession, but also among CAM representatives themselves. The Council was declared as having finished its work by the Ministry of Health, even though the social closure process of some of the therapies has not fully been completed. In 2015 the government finally published the legal requirements for setting up higher education degrees in acupuncture, osteopathy, chiropractic, naturopathy and phytotherapy through Directives 172-B-F/2015. However, the Directive excluded homeopathy and traditional Chinese medicine. The requirements for a homeopathic degree have yet to be published at the time of writing. Homeopathy is a controversial practice, as its philosophical principles are opposed to those of Western scientific medicine, and therefore not easily accepted by conventional medical practitioners – although there is a group of medical doctors who have practised homeopathy in Portugal (Almeida 2012). Interestingly, the requirements for establishing higher education degrees in traditional Chinese medicine were published in 2018, through Directive 45/2018. This takes such licensed therapies outside the formal realm of health support work as they have in effect achieved social closure.

Data show that there are 11 courses running in the country: 8 in osteopathy (the first BSc started in 2016–17) and 3 in acupuncture (the first BSc started in 2017–18), accredited by the A3ES (2019). At the same time, 13 course proposals submitted to the A3ES have been rejected, including for phytotherapy and naturopathy (Silva 2018). Osteopathy thus has been at the forefront of this regulation. According to A3ES, polytechnic schools should have a minimum of 60 per cent of permanent teaching staff and 15 per cent of teaching staff with a PhD on the subject being taught. For a course to be accredited, the A3ES also evaluates the proposed material resources and the qualifications of the course coordinator. Therefore setting up a CAM degree in the country has been challenging, as those who could be the providers of most of this teaching barely meet the qualification standards set by the A3ES (Silva 2018). Osteopathy, however, due to its close links to physiotherapy, has the benefit of having a teaching body borrowed from physiotherapy with the standard qualifications set out by the A3ES. Out of these 15 CAM courses accredited by the A3ES, only two run in public institutions, one in osteopathy in the Polytechnic Institute of Porto, and another in acupuncture, at the Polytechnic Institute of Setúbal. Other private institutions offering BSc degrees in acupuncture and/or osteopathy are the Piaget Institute, with schools in different parts of the country, the Atlantic University School of Health, and the Portuguese Red Cross, among others.

Such CAM practice, though, as in Brazil, remains marginalised – even though it has state legitimacy. This is underlined by the dislike by doctors of the appropriation of the word 'medicine' by CAM practices that are not Western scientific medicine. Accordingly, the introductory paragraph of Directive 45/2018 that underpins the licensure of, and educational arrangements for traditional Chinese medicine (TCM), states that to avoid potential misunderstanding between the present degree [in TCM] and the degree in medicine [scientific Western medicine], which is a university-exclusive degree, it is highlighted that TCM degree's marketing and promotional activities should be very clear about the type of teaching administered (Assembleia da República Portuguesa 2018: 902).

In this light, it is not surprising that in 2019, an anti-CAM manifesto, entitled 'For scientifically-based health practices', and signed by medical doctors, pharmacists, engineers, lawyers, among others, was submitted to Parliament. The manifesto requests that the government, among other things, revokes all the recent legislation on CAM regulation, as it has wrongly deceived the public into thinking CAM practices are effective (Carvalho 2019). Furthermore, the proponents of the Manifesto claim that CAM practices should be regulated, but not within the remit of health; rather, they should become part of the promotion of wellbeing. This anti-CAM manifesto was a response to a petition with several thousand signatures started early in 2019 for the integration of CAM in the SNS. This highlights the potentially transitory nature of the boundary between professionalised therapists and classically defined health support workers.

Alongside the statutory regulation of seven CAM professions, Western 'medical acupuncture' has become available to medical doctors exclusively as a postgraduate course since 2002. The course was proposed by the Portuguese Medical Society of Acupuncture (Sociedade Portuguesa Médica de Acupunctura, known as the SPMA) to the Portuguese Medical Council, who approved it. The SPMA was founded in August 2001 with the aim of promoting scientific research in medical acupuncture and supporting doctors who also practise Western medical acupuncture. There have been postgraduate courses in Western medical acupuncture since 2003 in the Abel Salazar's Biomedical Sciences Institute in Porto, since 2007 at the Faculty of Medicine in Coimbra, since 2010 in the Faculty of Medical Sciences at the New University of Lisbon, and since 2012 in the School of Medical Sciences at the University of Minho. There are also collaborations between the SPMA and other universities; among them is the University of Florianopolis, in Brazil. The key point here, though, is that again this medical enclave is not technically support work as it is ring fenced for the professionally qualified.

However, what can be classically classified as health support work, as in Brazil, is CAM practice that lies outside of these boundaries. In this respect, we need to particularly note the status and market position of CAM therapies which, although not statutorily regulated by Act 71/2013, have their own voluntary self-regulatory bodies. These include Ayurveda, aromatherapy, reiki and yoga, among others. For instance, the Portuguese Association for Ayurvedic Medicine is a voluntary association aiming to regulate Ayurvedic practice in the country. It is paralleled by the Portuguese Society of Aromatherapy, linked to the School of Aromatherapy, founded in 2009. Moreover, reiki therapy exists as support work too, overseen in part on a voluntary basis by the Portuguese Association of Reiki founded in 2008, with the aim of ethically informing practitioners and patients. There is also a multiplicity of yoga associations in the country – a practice that is far from integrated into the SNS. These exemplify the CAM practice areas where the greatest degree of marginality exists in Portugal and where the support work tag most appropriately fits, as it once did in the recent past for the seven CAM therapies that have now gained official legitimacy through the pioneering legislation that has underpinned their social closure (Almeida et al 2018a).

To sum up, CAM practitioners in Portugal have to a large degree been statutorily regulated, and the title of specialist in one of the seven CAM therapies has been protected by law. Medical doctors, however, have also practised Western medical acupuncture, and although homeopathy has not been regulated by the Medical Council, there are several doctors practising homeopathy in the country as well. Nonetheless, while the use of CAM within the SNS by the medically qualified is not significant and CAM as a practice remains fairly marginalised by orthodox medicine, there is still a large amount of CAM practice undertaken by therapists who can be defined as health support workers outside of those groups who have recently gained exclusionary social closure.

Conclusion

This chapter has outlined the status and market position of CAM practices and practitioners, especially with reference to the cases of Brazil and Portugal. In both countries, CAM demand, as well as state and medical interest in CAM, has increased. Both Brazilian and Portuguese states have created new legislation on CAM, and there is greater recognition of the contribution of these therapies for health and social care. As noted, such recognition has been expressed in different ways (see also Almeida et al 2018b). In terms of theories of professions, as has been seen, seven groups of CAM practitioners have obtained exclusionary closure backed by the state in Portugal, yet such professions have limited power as they operate mostly outside the public health system, are paid directly by the service user and are not widely available through the SNS. Furthermore, not all of these CAM therapies have made it to the higher education system yet. Osteopathy and acupuncture have been at the forefront of CAM regulation in the country, as they are the only ones with degree programmes accredited by the state and running in both public and private higher education institutions. Therefore even the few CAM occupations that have gained statutory regulation are in a liminal state and have not fully achieved visibility and the standards set out by law 71/2013. As President Sousa suggested in vetoing the governmental proposal recognising the setting up of the School of Non-Conventional Therapeutics, osteopathy and acupuncture courses are 'under experimentation' in the country (Presidência da República 2019). This accentuates the marginality of those CAM support workers who lie outside the professional and educational system. Here homeopathy in particular remains in limbo as it is the only mainstream CAM therapy still waiting for the government to publish the requirements for setting up higher education degrees and therefore the social closure process is not yet complete.

In Brazil, in turn, 29 CAM therapies have been regulated to be practised by primary health care professionals, including community health workers, within the SUS. Contrary to Portugal, in Brazil CAM therapies are widely used within the SUS. Yet it has been suggested that the visibility and recognition of these therapies within the SUS have been low (Barros et al 2018). CAM practice within the multidisciplinary teams of the ESF generates conflict among team members, puts pressure on their workloads and is secondary to biomedical consultations and treatments. Another main aspect of the Brazilian state is that it supports CAM therapies without recognising CAM therapists; CAM is therefore seen as a complementary resource used by different primary care professionals including medical doctors, within a multi-professional team. Medically qualified practitioners have acquired their voluntary training and qualification in one or another form of CAM usually through postgraduate courses run by their professional associations. CAM practices outside the SUS are not regulated and therefore have operated with voluntary forms of self-regulation, such as association membership – thus enabling this aspect of their operation to be quintessentially seen as health support work.

What makes the Brazilian and the Portuguese cases interesting is that, despite implementing different CAM policies, CAM practices and practitioners have a shared common status and position in health care in both countries. The Portuguese case suggests a hierarchy within the health care division of labour and within the education system too. Within the education system, courses in specific CAM therapies have been regulated to operate within the polytechnic teaching institutions, differently from the medical profession, which has university-exclusive teaching. CAM practitioners remain marginalised within health care, with limited power, autonomy and control over their knowledge and practice, and with educational standards set out by the state. By entering the higher education system, they must comply with standardised protocols and curricula aligned with the 'scientific' medical profession (Welsh et al 2004) – with the educational standards for each of the CAM therapies supported by the government including disciplines such as anatomy and pathology. While formally professionalised, in the same way as non-professionalised health support workers, the favoured seven CAM therapists are subordinated to, and undervalued by, more orthodox health care professions.

In the case of Brazil too, many CAM practitioners are marginal to the health system, as they lack statutory regulation, and therefore are excluded from the mainstream health care workforce. In the same way as many support workers, they lack mandatory registers and state accreditation. CAM as a therapy, however, has entered the Brazilian health care system in a very substantial way, particularly as used by a variety of primary health care professionals, including medical doctors, nurses, dentists, and community health workers – the latter of whom contribute to a broader perspective on health care, including biomedical as well as psycho-social dimensions. Professionalised community health workers – like support workers – often feel discontentment over their work conditions, though, due to inadequate infrastructure and the lack of enthusiasm about their role among other members of the ESF's multi-professional teams (Barros et al 2018), in which they have become optional in the health care division of labour.

Furthermore, both Brazilian and Portuguese cases illustrate well the complexity of the term CAM, similar to the 'support worker' definition. A main characteristic of definitions of CAM and support work has been their lack of state support and state regulation. Defining CAM or general support work primarily according to its lack of mandatory statutory regulation thus can become problematic, given recent state involvement in CAM regulation, as illustrated by the Brazilian and Portuguese cases. State recognition, however, does not necessarily mean that CAM practitioners have improved their status, as shown by the situation in Portugal because they are marginalised within the health care division of labour, when compared to other health professionals. At the same time, both support workers and health professionals involved with CAM play a crucial, yet often invisible, role in dealing with the increasing levels of vulnerability of an ageing population with multiple needs. Here they have the virtue of focusing on spending more time with the service user compared to orthodox health professionals in societies necessarily ever more centred on care.

References

Agência de Avaliação e Acreditação do Ensino Superior (2019) Acreditação de Ciclo de Estudos, www.a3es.pt/pt/acreditacao-e-auditoria/resultados-dos-processos-de-acreditacao/acreditacao-de-ciclos-de-estudos

Almeida, J. (2012) 'The differential incorporation of CAM into the medical establishment: The case of acupuncture and homeopathy in Portugal', *Health Sociology Review* 21(1): 5–22.

Almeida, J. and Gabe, J. (2016) 'CAM within a field force of countervailing powers: The case of Portugal', *Social Science and Medicine* 155: 73–81.

Almeida, J., Siegel, P. and Barros, N.F. (2018a) 'Governing complementary and alternative medicine in Brazil and Portugal: Implications for CAM professionals and the public', in Chamberlain, J.M., Dent, M. and Saks, M. (eds) *Professional Health Regulation in the Public Interest: International Perspectives*, Bristol: Policy Press.

Almeida, J., Siegel, P. and Barros, N.F. (2018b) 'Towards the glocalisation of complementary and alternative medicine: Homeopathy, acupuncture and Traditional Chinese medicine practice and regulation in Brazil and Portugal', in Brosnan, C., Vuolanto, P. and Danell, J.B. (eds) *Complementary and Alternative Medicine: Knowledge Production and Social Transformation*, Basingstoke: Palgrave Macmillan.

Assembleia da República Portuguesa (2013) 'Lei n° 71/2013 de 2 de setembro: Regulamenta a Lei n° 45/2003, de 22 de agosto, relativamente ao exercício profissional das atividades de aplicação de terapêuticas não convencionais', in *Diário da República* n° 168/2013, Série I de 2013-09-02, https://dre.pt/application/conteudo/499569

Assembleia da República Portuguesa (2018) 'Portaria n° 45/2018 de 9 de fevereiro', in *Diário da República* n° 29, Série I de 2018-02-09, https://dre.pt/application/file/a/114665489

Barros N.F., Oliveira, M.C.S., Ferreira, F.C. and Gomes, T.C. (2016) 'Práticas Integrativas e Complementares na Atenção Primária em Saúde: a implementação de um modelo complementar precário', *III Congreso de Estudios Poscoloniales y IV Jornadas de Feminismo Poscolonial: Interrupciones desde el Sur: Habitando Cuerpos, Territorios y Saberes*, 12–15 December, Buenos Aires, Argentina.

Barros, N.F., Spadacio, C. and Costa, M.V. (2018) 'Trabalho interprofissional e as práticas integrativas e complementares no contexto da antenção primária à saúde: potenciais e desafios', *Saúde Debate* 42(1): 163–73.

Brazilian Ministry of Health (2011) *Portaria nº 719*, Diário Oficial da União – Seção 1, 7 April, www.conselho.saude.pr.gov.br/arquivos/File/Conferencias/10%20CES/PROGRA01.PDF

Brazilian Ministry of Health (2017a) *Portaria nº 849*, Gabinete do Ministro, 27 March, http://bvsms.saude.gov.br/bvs/saudelegis/gm/2017/prt0849_28_03_2017.html

Brazilian Ministry of Health (2017b) 'Ministério da Saúde inclui 14 novos procedimentos na Política Nacional de Práticas Integrativas', http://portalms.saude.gov.br/noticias/agencia-saude/27929-ministerio-da-saude-inclui-14-novos-procedimentos-na-politica-nacional-de-praticas-integrativas

Brazilian Ministry of Health (2017c) *Portaria nº 2.436*, Gabinete de Ministro, 21 September, http://bvsms.saude.gov.br/bvs/saudelegis/gm/2017/prt2436_22_09_2017.html

Brazilian Ministry of Health (2018) *Portaria nº 702*, Gabinete do Ministro, 21 March, http://bvsms.saude.gov.br/bvs/saudelegis/gm/2018/prt0702_22_03_2018.html

Brazilian Ministry of Health (2019) 'Práticas integrativas e complementares (PICS): quais são e para que servem', http://portalms.saude.gov.br/saude-de-a-z/praticas-integrativas-e-complementares

British Medical Acupuncture Society (2019) 'Who are the BMAS?', www.medical-acupuncture.co.uk/

Cant, S. and Sharma, U. (1996) 'Demarcation and transformation within homoeopathic knowledge. A strategy of professionalisation', *Social Science and Medicine* 42(4): 579–88.

Carvalho, P. (2019) 'Manifesto contra "retrocesso civilizacional" das terapêuticas não convencionais entregue no Parlamento', *Público*, 26 March, www.publico.pt/2019/03/26/sociedade/noticia/manifesto-retrocesso-civilizacional-terapeuticas-nao-convencionais-1866895

Cavendish, C. (2013) *An Independent Review into Healthcare Assistants and Support Workers in the NHS and Social Care Settings*, https://assets.publishing.service.gov.uk/government/uploads/system/uploads/attachment_data/file/236212/Cavendish_Review.pdf

Comissão Nacional de Práticas Integrativas e Complementares em Saúde (2018) *Auriculoterapia. Informativo Bimestral da CNPICS*, 1st edition, 08/2018, http://189.28.128.100/dab/docs/portaldab/documentos/informes/Informativo_PICS_bimestral_1ed_08_2018.pdf

Durão, A.V.R. and Menezes, C.A.F. (2016) 'Na esteira de E.P. Thompson: relações sociais de género e o fazer-se agente comunitária de saúde no município do Rio de Janeiro', *Trabalho, Educação e Saúde* 14(2): 355–76.

Halpern, S.A. (1990) 'Medicalization as professional process: Postwar trends in pediatrics', *Journal of Health and Social Behavior* 31(1): 28–42.

Harris, M. and Haines, A. (2010) 'Brazil's family health programme', *British Medical Journal* 341: c4945.

Health Education England (2015) *Raising the Bar: Shape of Caring: A Review of the Future Education and Training of Registered Nurses and Care Assistants*, London: HEE.

House of Commons (2010) *Science and Technology Committee – Fourth Report Evidence Check 2: Homeopathy*, https://publications.parliament.uk/pa/cm200910/cmselect/cmsctech/45/4502.htm

Ijaz, N., Boon, H., Muzzin, L. and Welsh, S. (2016) 'State risk discourse and the regulatory preservation of traditional medicine knowledge: The case of acupuncture in Ontario, Canada', *Social Science and Medicine* 170: 97–105.

Kelner, M., Wellman, B., Boon, H. and Welsh, S. (2004) 'Responses of established healthcare to the professionalization of complementary and alternative medicine in Ontario', *Social Science and Medicine* 59: 915–30.

Levy, L. (1966) 'Factors which facilitate or impede transfer of medical functions from physicians to paramedical personnel', *Journal of Health and Human Behavior* 7(1): 50–54.

Manthorpe, J. and Martineau, S. (2008) *Support Workers: Their Role and Tasks: A Scoping Review*, London: King's College.

NHS England and NHS Clinical Commissioners (2017) 'Items which should not routinely be prescribed in primary care: Guidance for CCGs', www.england.nhs.uk/wp-content/uploads/2017/11/items-which-should-not-be-routinely-precscribed-in-pc-ccg-guidance.pdf

NHS Health Careers (2019) 'Clinical support staff', www.healthcareers.nhs.uk/explore-roles/wider-healthcare-team/roles-wider-healthcare-team/clinical-support-staff

National Institute for Health and Care Excellence (2016) *Low Back Pain and Sciatica in over 16s: Assessment and Management*, NICE guideline 30 November, www.nice.org.uk/guidance/ng59

Oliveira, M.C.S. (2018) 'As (in)visibilidades do Lian Gong na atenção primária em saúde', MSc Collective Health, Faculty of Medical Sciences, State University of Campinas, São Paulo, Brazil (unpublished).

Polich, G., Dole, C. and Kaptchuk, T.J. (2010) 'The need to act a little more "scientific": Biomedical researchers investigating complementary and alternative medicine', *Sociology of Health and Illness* 32(1): 106–22.

Presidência da República (2019) *Presidente da República devolve Diploma ao Governo*, www.presidencia.pt/?idc=10&idi=159777

Saks, M. (1995) *Professions and the Public Interest: Medical Power, Altruism and Alternative Medicine*, London: Routledge.

Saks, M. (1996) 'From quackery to complementary medicine: The shifting boundaries between orthodox and unorthodox medical knowledge', in Cant, S. and Sharma, U. (eds) *Complementary and Alternative Medicines: Knowledge in Practice*, London: Free Association Books.

Saks, M. (2008) 'Policy dynamics: Marginal groups in the healthcare division of labour', in Kuhlmann, E. and Saks, M. (eds) *Rethinking Professional Governance: International Directions in Healthcare*, Bristol: Policy Press.

Saks, M. (2015) 'Inequalities, marginality and the professions', *Current Sociology Review* 63(6): 850–68.

Sarre, S., Maben, J., Aldus, C., Schneider, J., Wharrad, H., Nicholson, C. and Arthur, A. (2018) 'The challenges of training, support and assessment of healthcare support workers: A qualitative study of experiences in three English acute hospitals', *International Journal of Nursing Studies* 79: 145–53.

Siahpush, M. (1999) 'A critical review of the sociology of alternative medicine: Research on users, practitioners and the orthodoxy', *Health* 4(2): 159–78.

Silva, S. (2018) 'Já foram autorizadas 15 licenciaturas em terapias alternativas em Portugal. Ensino Superior', *Jornal O Público*, www.publico.pt/2018/03/26/sociedade/noticia/ja-foram-autorizadas-15-licenciaturas-em-terapias-alternativas-em-portugal-1808005

Sociedade Internacional de Terapia (2016) *Conceitos Gerais*, www.sinte.com.br/faq/index.php?action=artikel&cat=14&id=96&artlang=pt-br

Tesser, C.D., Moré, A.O.O., Santos, M.C., da Silva, E.D.C., Farias, F.T.P. and Botelho, L.J. (2019) 'Auriculotherapy in primary health care: A large-scale educational experience in Brazil', *Journal of Integrative Medicine* 17(4): 302–309.

Welsh, S., Kelner, M., Wellman, B. and Boon, H. (2004) 'Moving forward? Complementary and alternative practitioners seeking self-regulation', *Sociology of Health and Illness* 26(2): 216–41.

Wiese, M., Oster, C. and Pincombe, J. (2010) 'Understanding the emerging relationship between complementary medicine and mainstream health care: A review of the literature', *Health* 14: 326–42.

Witz, A. (1992) *Professions and Patriarchy*, London: Routledge.

World Health Organization (2013) *WHO Traditional Medicine Strategy: 2014–2023*, WHO: Geneva.

TEN

Personal support workers and the labour market

Audrey Laporte, Adrian Rohit Dass, Whitney Berta,
Raisa Deber and Katherine Zagrodney

Introduction

Personal support workers (PSWs) represent a significant portion of the health care labour force in many countries. Using the example of Canada, this chapter focuses on the PSW labour market and its relationship to supply characteristics. Since the PSW labour market is situated within the broader health care labour market, in which professional and occupational dynamics, competition among various occupations and related hierarchies, and professional exclusionary closure operate (Saks 2010), it is considered within this context, in line with a neo-Weberian approach. PSWs are generally best classified under the working class in accordance with Weberian theory, wherein their key asset is labour power as opposed to formal credentials (Weber 1968). Given their shared position within this larger health care labour market, individuals making up the PSW labour force are likely to possess common traits and face similar barriers to economic mobility opportunities. Such shared characteristics among PSWs may lead to the inability to secure employment in other more valued (monetary and otherwise) health care occupations with higher educational requirements (such as nursing), resulting in PSW employment as a default option for some of these individuals. We largely focus on the Canadian PSW labour market in this chapter, but such factors apply to many PSWs in a wider global context.

This chapter begins with a general description of the importance of the PSW labour market, and includes a definition of PSWs. It explores past, current, and forecasted supply and demand. Key contextual factors, including regulatory models in Canada, are noted. Since the data suggests that the PSW labour market is better thought of as a series of sub-markets which tend to differ along the lines of such factors as wages and hours worked, the analysis includes differences by sector across a multitude of individual and job characteristics, as well as labour market outcomes. It then examines individual characteristics such as socio-demographics (gender, age, marital status, immigrant status, visible minority status, ethnicity, Aboriginal status), family and household characteristics (informal care giving variables, family member employment), health status (self-reported health, injury rates and severity, disability, medical conditions), and education and training variables (highest level of education, relevance of education, years of experience). It next describes PSW job characteristics and how these affect labour market outcomes, including work status (full-time, part-time and casual status, as well as schedule and shift types), hours worked, wages, unionisation, benefits and pensions. Relevant differences by location (by province and urban versus rural) are also described where data are available.

The importance of the labour market for personal support workers

Defining personal support workers

PSWs are frontline non-professionalised health care workers who provide care to a large variety of health care users, where care tasks typically involve helping patients with activities of daily living, in addition to performing more medically-inclined tasks (Lum et al 2015). PSWs are referred to under a large array of titles – from health care aides to nursing assistants. PSWs work across a range of health care settings, which are commonly divided into three sectors: nursing homes or long-term care homes, home and community, and hospitals (Health Professions Regulatory Advisory Council 2006). Within the PSW labour market, there is a great amount of heterogeneity by sector and work location. Differences may exist in tasks performed, title usage, forms of regulation, education, skill level and mix, job characteristics, individual and socio-demographic characteristics. Such sectoral and geographic discrepancies may constrain job mobility across sectors, which could have important implications for health human resource planning.

Health care can be delivered to a variety of patients in a multitude of ways. In Canada, as in many other countries, demand has increased due to changes in patient demographics – such as an ageing population and a higher proportion of patients with chronic conditions (Roberts et al 2015). Since the cost of delivering care often varies across care sectors, there is increasing pressure to shift the site of health care delivery from hospitals to the home and community sector (Health Professions Regulatory Advisory Council 2006), which is presumed to be less expensive, and to place greater reliance on PSWs as a lower cost option for care delivery (Canadian Home Care Association 2008).

Supply and demand for personal support workers: past, current and forecast

In Canada, national census data shows the number of individuals working in 'assisting occupations in support of health services' (which includes PSWs under such titles as nurse aides) has more than doubled from 165,385 in 1996 to 346,880 in 2016 (Statistics Canada 1996, 2016). The same source reports that the number of nurses increased from 246,800 in 1996 to 327,780 in 2006. To the extent that these data accurately capture the workforce, the proportion of PSW-type positions in the total professional nursing and assisted occupations grew from 40 per cent in 1996 to 51 per cent in 2016. An additional complexity is that there are several categories of nurses in Canada. Registered Nurses (RNs) must usually complete four years of university education; Licensed Practical Nurse (LPNs), called Registered Practical Nurses (RPNs) in Ontario, usually require only two years of college education (National Nursing Assessment Service 2018). RNs in most provinces have a broader scope of practice, including tasks which LPNs and PSWs would not be permitted to perform. While PSW employment rates increased by approximately 63 per cent between 1995 and 2003, RN employment only increased by just over 7 per cent, and LPN employment declined by close to 22 per cent (Pyper 2004).

PSWs often work in concert with other health care providers such as nurses, as well as with informal, typically unpaid caregivers, both in a complementary capacity and as substitutes for nurses to deal with less complex tasks and/or patients. In Canada's long-term care sector, nurses have largely shifted to a management and oversight role and have increasingly been replaced by PSWs in the delivery of direct care (Berta et al 2013). Similarly, in the home and community sector, the proportion of paid home care workers who were PSWs increased from approximately 38 per cent in 1999 to 66 per cent in 2003 (Pyper 2004). However, capturing PSW data is a challenge, and these trends may reflect improvements in encapsulating the PSW population, as well as actual growth over time. The rising importance of PSWs in the delivery of care is projected to continue in Canada (Canadian Occupational Projection System 2017b). Alberta Health Services forecast demand for 3,264 additional PSWs by the year 2020, which represents a doubling over ten years (Bloom et al 2012). Moreover, total yearly hours and the number of full-time equivalent (FTE) PSWs in Manitoba's home and community sector was expected to almost double by 2037, by adding approximately 90–100 additional FTE PSWs each year in addition to filling vacant positions where vacancy rates were between 8 and 10 per cent (Minister of Health Seniors and Active Living 2016). Other countries have also projected increases in the demand for PSWs, including the United States (Bureau of Labor Statistics, 2015), Ireland (Behan et al 2009) and Japan (Aoki 2016).

Forecasts for Canada over the period 2017–26 suggest that the overall supply of PSW and related occupations will be sufficient to meet demand (Department of Employment and Social Development Canada 2018). However, multiple provincial and sector-specific projections have anticipated that there may be inadequate supply in certain regions or sub-sectors, particularly in home and community care. One projection showed a large gap between the number of health care users that would require PSW care and the number of PSWs available to provide care, which was estimated to expand from a ratio of one PSW to 17 health care recipients in 2001 to one to 45 by 2046 (Home Care Sector Study Corporation 2003). Although discrepancies exist in projections between future demand and supply of PSWs, there are also indications of an already existing shortage of PSWs working in home and community and long-term care. PSW retention and recruitment are considered major challenges in health care delivery across the Organisation for Economic Co-operation and Development countries (Canadian Home Care Association 2008; Fujisawa and Colombo 2009). Reasons include recruitment difficulties (Sims-Gould et al 2010) and high turnover within the PSW labour market, especially in the home and community sector (Denton et al 2006).

Multiple factors may affect recruitment and retention of PSWs in different sectors. These factors include job satisfaction, flexibility of schedules, wages and other job characteristics (Keefe et al 2011; Sims-Gould et al 2010), as well as socio-demographic and individual characteristics. These characteristics can influence decisions to work, hours worked and the choice of sector. For example, Canadian Occupational Projection System (2017a, 2017b) data indicates that the proportion of immigrants expected to fill PSW-related occupations in the home and community sector are much higher (39 per cent) than for hospital and long-term care (16 per cent). Furthermore, it is anticipated that PSWs shifting between sectors will result in 40 per cent of long-term care and hospital positions being filled by PSWs currently working in the home and community sector. In contrast, only 21 per cent of PSW positions in this latter sector are expected to be filled by individuals working in other occupations (primarily home-based child care), and to a lesser extent by immigrants and new job seekers. There is no indication of hospital or long-term care PSWs filling home and community roles. Moreover, some of the sectoral differences in supply and demand are complicated by the fact that supply from the less attractive home and community sector is anticipated to fill demand in the long-term care and hospital sectors.

Contextual factors of potential influence on the supply of personal support workers

Domestic regulations

Regulations for health care occupations which restrict who can work in different job positions are important contextual factors that influence supply within a given labour market. One key distinction is whether a provider is designated as a profession. Since health care in Canada is under provincial/territorial jurisdiction, such governments determine which occupations are so designated. However, they tend to delegate responsibility to self-governing regulatory bodies (often called Colleges) wherein members of the profession decide on the skills and knowledge requirements to belong to a given profession, set standards of practice, and offer a venue to assess and discipline members to protect the public's interest (Zelisko et al 2014). Health professionals must be licensed by their provincial/territorial regulatory college in order to practice in that jurisdiction. Governments may also specify 'controlled acts' which can only be performed by regulated professionals, although in some cases these can be delegated to others if the regulated professional supervises them. These are often specified in provincial legislation as standards; examples include New Brunswick's Home Support Service Standards (2011), Alberta's Long-term Care Accommodations Standards and Checklist (2010), and Ontario's Long-Term Care Homes Act (2007). Unlike doctors and nurses, who are regulated in all Canadian provinces, PSWs are not in a regulated profession – although the province of Quebec does allow PSWs to choose to become a 'voluntary professional' under the title 'home health attendant' (Government of Quebec 2016).

However, PSWs may be subject to some regulatory controls to the extent that they perform controlled acts. PSWs can also be subject to a provincial registry. Registries can be voluntary or compulsory, and serve multiple purposes – including providing PSWs with career opportunities. Nonetheless, they often seek to protect vulnerable patient populations by imposing a minimum entry to practice requirement on PSWs and by requiring employers to report any alleged abuse to the Registry (Foerster and Murtagh 2013). Registries can impact supply of a labour market in a variety of ways – for instance, as a barrier to supply if registration is viewed as increasing the level of difficulty to enter the profession, or, alternatively, registration could potentially increase supply if it serves as a source of recognition and legitimacy for an occupation. At the time of writing, three Canadian provinces had established PSW registries: British Columbia, Nova Scotia and Ontario. For examples of PSW regulation in the UK, as well as more details on the potential risks to the public as a result of the general lack of PSW regulation, see Chapter five of this volume.

The expansion of home and community and institutional long-term care sectors

The expansion of care delivery in home and community and long-term care settings is a result of multiple factors, including an ageing population (Health Council of Canada 2012) that has expressed a desire to age in place (Carstairs and Keon 2007), and technological advances which make it easier to deliver care in the home and community sector. A number of provincial initiatives have encouraged the shift in care from hospitals to this sector. One related complexity is that health care in Canada is organised on a provincial/territorial basis. Since the Canada Health Act requires public payment only for medically necessary care if delivered in hospitals or by physicians (Deber 2018), provincial plans can choose whether and to what extent to pay for care delivered in the home and community or long-term care sectors, but are not required to do so, meaning that patients (or their private insurers) may have to meet much of the costs of such care. Greater emphasis on the home and community sector has increased demand for PSWs to provide direct home making and social care services. Previous work reported that 70–80 per cent of home and community care in Canada was provided by PSWs (Home Care Sector Study Corporation 2003), which meant cost savings to management, given the nursing shortage and rising nursing wages (Rhéaume et al 2007). Accordingly, the PSW labour market must be examined in relation to the supply and demand for other related health care workers.

Wages and hours worked

Wages

Wages are an important component in the study of a given labour market. Over the years 1993–2010, average PSW wages across Canada were C$14.00 per hour (adjusted to year 2006), as compared to the provincial minimum wage in 2006 of C$6.50–7.75 per hour (Department of Employment and Social Development Canada 2017a, 2017b). Although PSW hourly wages increased slightly from C$14.44 in 1997 to C$14.60 in 2003, LPN wages declined slightly from C$19.00 to C$18.89 while RN hourly wages increased from C$23.97 to C$26.13 over the same time period (Pyper 2004). The slight decline in LPN wage levels observed in Canada over time may be a result of LPNs being replaced by the generally less expensive PSWs, resulting in the LPN wage moving toward PSW wage rates in order to remain competitive (Zarnett et al 2009). At the same time, RN wages may have increased as PSWs take on a greater proportion of the lower skilled tasks, leaving RNs to perform the higher-skilled tasks. In this regard, PSWs have been found to earn the lowest hourly wages of 16 health-related occupations (including various health care professions and administrative roles) (Tijdens et al 2013). Most of these other providers are members of regulated professions that require higher levels of education and training and carry out different tasks.

Another factor likely to influence these trends in wages by occupation is differential movement between sectors; since wages differ by sector, differences in the proportion of workers in these sectors over time could result in changes in average wages earned for each occupation (Montgomery et al 2005). For example, in 2016–17 personal support aides (the group including PSWs working in hospitals and long-term care) had a median hourly wage of C$20.00 whereas the median wage for PSWs in home support was C$15.80 (Department of Employment and Social Development Canada 2017a, 2017b). Features that are inherent to each sector – such as the differences in unionisation rates and size of workplace – are likely to impact such sectoral differences in wages (Baughman and Smith 2008; Montgomery et al 2005). PSW wages not only differ by sector, but also by province (Department of Employment and Social Development Canada 2017a, 2017b). Some of these PSW wage discrepancies are attributable to differences in minimum wages, average working wages, living costs by province, and overtime. PSWs in the Eastern Canadian provinces tend to have the lowest wages (Home Care Sector Study Corporation 2003; Korczyk 2004) corresponding in part to the lower per capita income in these provinces compared to other parts of the country. However, province-specific strategies can also affect PSW wages. For instance, one province (Ontario) announced a specific wage increase strategy for PSWs with a goal of a C$16.50 per hour minimum by 1 April 2016 (Ministry of Health and Long-term Care 2015), as compared to the minimum wage for the province of C$11.25 per hour.

Most provincial reports also show a wide range of PSW wages within provinces (Sims-Gould et al 2010). Rural PSWs often receive lower wages than urban PSWs (Baughman and Smith 2008; Price-Glynn and Rakovski 2012), reflecting in part variations in the cost of living between urban and rural locations, but also the distribution across sectors. In urban areas PSWs are more likely to work in hospitals (Montgomery et al 2005) whereas PSWs in rural areas are more likely to work in home and community care (Dill et al 2012). The impact of wages, demographics, and other characteristics on the number of hours worked by PSWs are now discussed.

Number of hours worked

Internationally, the average total PSW hours worked per year range from approximately 611 to 1,786 hours, with weekly hours worked ranging from 13 to 38 hours (Hewko et al 2015). The average number of hours PSWs work by sector also varies, but the literature differs as to which sectors are associated with the most hours. Some Canadian sources report that PSWs in home and community work approximately 30 hours per week or less (Home Care Sector Study Corporation 2003; Zeytinoglu et al 2016), but other sources suggest they tend to work more than 40 hours per week (Dill et al 2012). Discrepancies in reported hours worked by sector are related to what is counted as hours worked; PSWs in home and community may be more likely to have unpaid hours of work resulting from a lack of appropriate allotted hours per patient leading to additional unpaid hours of work provided by PSWs to meet patient needs, unpaid planning and preparation time, and travel time between clients (Home Care Sector Study Corporation 2003). Differences in year-round PSW participation by sector may also occur, as PSWs in home and community are the least likely to work year round as compared to PSWs in long-term care or hospitals (Montgomery et al 2005).

Individual characteristics and the relationship to labour market outcomes

Socio-demographics

The PSW workforce in Canada is largely comprised of women (Dill et al 2012; Lum et al 2015; Sims-Gould et al 2010; Zeytinoglu et al 2016) as it is in many others countries such as Australia, Denmark, France and The Netherlands (Korczyk 2004). Extending recruitment to target men is a potential future strategy to fill PSW positions, although men may be more costly to employ if they have a greater set of alternative jobs offering higher pay (Hegewisch and Liepmann 2010). It is worth noting that the proportion of females working as PSWs in Canada from 1993 to 2010 significantly differed by sector: PSWs in home and community (90.6 per cent) and long-term care (89.5 per cent) had higher proportions of female PSWs as compared to hospital PSWs (66.3 per cent) (Zagrodney et al 2019). Although long-term care PSWs often have similar proportions of females to PSWs in the home and community sector, the latter frequently report the highest averages overall of female PSWs in Canada (Canadian Occupational Projection System 2018; Dill et al 2012) and the United States (Montgomery et al 2005).

PSWs also generally constitute an older workforce than RNs, LPNs and other health professionals (Home Care Sector Study Corporation 2003), as well as in comparison to the general labour market (Korczyk 2004). In a nationwide sample of PSWs for 1993–2010, home and community PSWs were significantly older than hospital PSWs, while long-term PSWs were the youngest. However, although these differences were statistically significant, they were small, with average ages approximately 41 for long-term care, 42 for hospital, and 43 years for PSWs working in home and community settings. Nonetheless, there were more PSWs over the age of 50 than under the age of 30, with the average age of PSWs significantly increasing over time (Zagrodney et al 2019). Potential reasons for an older PSW workforce include better retention of PSWs who continue to work into older age, a decline in recruitment of younger individuals and/or an increase in recruitment of older individuals into the PSW workforce. The limited inflow of young PSWs entering the PSW labour market raises concerns about the long run sustainability of PSW supply. Younger PSWs typically work for lower wages (Baughman and Smith 2008; Price-Glynn and Rakovski 2012), but may also provide fewer hours of work, particularly if they also have family care giving responsibilities (Alamgir et al

2008). Projections are that the majority (72 per cent) of employment opportunities from 2017 to 2026 for home and community PSW-type jobs are expected to open up as a result of retirements (Canadian Occupational Protection System 2017a), with comparatively fewer employment opportunities (44 per cent) expected to emerge from retirements in the long-term care and hospital sectors (Canadian Occupational Projection System 2017b). Whether PSW supply will be able to meet the demands in home and community as many PSWs retire in this sector is uncertain.

As in other countries, immigrants have traditionally been a major source of labour supply for PSW-type work in Canada. The proportions of PSWs with immigrant status are high in comparison to the general working population in Canada (Minister of Health Seniors and Active Living 2016; Montgomery et al 2005; Sims–Gould et al 2010; Zeytinoglu et al 2016). The proportion of immigrants working as PSWs has increased over time in the period 1993–2010 (Zagrodney et al 2019). One possible reason for relatively high proportions of immigrant PSWs is the difficulties encountered by foreign-trained nurses in attaining registration in most Canadian jurisdictions. The characteristics of immigrant PSWs such as age and education level are underreported in the current literature and require further investigation. As mentioned earlier, there are anticipated differences in the proportions of immigrant PSWs by sector. In the home and community sector and in certain Canadian provinces (British Columbia and Ontario), the proportion of immigrants found in PSW samples have been as high as 47 per cent (Sims–Gould et al 2010) as opposed to only 16 per cent projected in both long-term care and hospital sectors nationally (Canadian Occupational Projection System 2017b). Ethnicity, visible minority status, and 'race' are often studied together in the PSW literature. In Canada a larger proportion of PSWs are visible minorities in comparison to the general working population, especially within the home and community sector (Lum et al 2015). In the United States, ethnicity and 'race' have been found to be significant predictors of working in full-time PSW positions (Potter et al 2006) and PSW wage levels (Price-Glynn and Rakovski 2012). In Canada the proportion of home and community PSWs with Aboriginal status was 4.8 per cent over the period 1993–2010 (Zagrodney et al 2019) which was higher than the proportion in the general working population of 3.5 per cent in 2006 (Statistics Canada 2006).

Marital status may also influence supply to the extent that a partner's labour force status, income, and hours worked impacts the labour market behaviours of PSWs. The majority (approximately 60–70 per cent) of PSWs in Canadian samples are married or living in common-law relationships (Dill et al 2012; Zeytinoglu et al 2016), although this may vary by location within the country. A Canada-wide sample shows no significant differences in marital status by sector (Zagrodney et al 2019). Marital status, though, has been shown to correlate with the wages and hours worked by PSWs, with married PSWs receiving up to 5 per cent higher wages than non-married PSWs (Baughman and Smith 2008) and single PSWs working fewer hours on average than married PSWs or those in common-law relationships (Potter et al 2006).

Family and household characteristics

Since PSWs are a workforce largely comprised of women, and female PSWs provide more informal care outside of work on average than men, PSW supply is affected by family and household characteristics that include informal care giving for their children and older family members (Price-Glynn and Rakovski 2012). Approximately half of PSWs in Canada reported living with children (Dill et al 2012), following a common international pattern (Hewko et al 2015). Sector differences in terms of flexibility in work hours and scheduling may facilitate or hinder the ability of PSWs to participate in the labour market given other responsibilities related to the family and household. PSWs in long-term care were significantly more likely to live with children and pre-school aged children than were home and community or hospital PSWs (Zagrodney et al 2019). Other family characteristics such as living with a family member with a disability are expected to similarly impact labour supply behaviours, as approximately one-third of a sample of Canadian PSWs reported living with at least one family member over the age of 16 with a disability.

Family and household employment may also impact the labour supply behaviours of PSWs. For instance, PSWs may increase their hours worked out of necessity in order to financially support unemployed family members. Zagrodney and colleagues (2019) found that approximately 47 per cent of PSWs were the major income earners in their household and that 26 per cent had one or more unemployed family members in their household. Statistically significant differences in unemployment for family members by sector were found, with hospital PSWs having the lowest prevalence of unemployed members within the family versus PSWs working in home and community or long-term care settings. In their study, family members of hospital PSWs were also significantly more likely to be employed full-year full time as compared to long-term care or home and community PSW family members.

Health status

Health status affects ability to work and PSW health has been found to be positively correlated with wages (Hamadi et al 2016). Measurements used to assess PSW health have included self-reported health status, injury severity and disability status, as well as the number and type of medical conditions. Compared to LPNs and/or RNs, PSWs generally have lower health scores across all of these health measures and are more likely to develop a disability that prevents them from working (Alamgir et al 2007, 2008; Baughman and Smith 2012). These differences are likely to be related to such job characteristics as skills, training, education and tasks performed. Musculoskeletal injuries accounted for up to 83 per cent of all PSW injuries in a Canadian sample and were more commonly reported in home and community and long-term care than in hospital (Alamgir et al 2007, 2008). Canadian PSWs working in home and community settings typically report significantly worse health than hospital or long-term care PSWs on a variety of health measures such as self-reported health and disability status (Zagrodney et al 2019).

The relationship between health and hours worked is complex because health may impact hours worked, while the number of hours worked may also impact health. Research suggests that casual or part-time PSWs are less likely to obtain a workplace injury or musculoskeletal injury than full-time PSWs. However, gender differences in health outcomes based on hours of work have also been reported (Alamgir et al 2008). Timing of hours worked may also influence PSW health; working non-standard hours (part-time or casual) correlated with worsened health status as measured by stress symptoms in a Canadian sample of PSWs working in home and community contexts (Zeytinoglu et al 2014). The comparatively low average health status and high injury rate among PSWs is a potential problem for their supply, given the relationship between health and labour supply.

Education and training levels

There are no nationwide education requirements for PSWs in Canada. A nationwide sample of PSWs from 1993 to 2010 found that 62.9 per cent of PSWs had at least a high school diploma or some post-secondary education without a certificate (Zagrodney et al 2019). Significant sectoral differences in education levels were found, whereby PSWs in long-term care generally had higher average educational attainment of a high school certificate or some post-secondary education without a certificate (66.5 per cent) than those working in home and community (61.4 per cent) or hospital (57.2 per cent) settings. A previous scoping international review (Hewko et al 2015) found a larger degree of variance in education levels, in which the percentage of PSWs with at least some post-secondary education ranged from 8 per cent in home and community or long-term care to 38.7 per cent in a hospital setting.

Differences in PSW education levels by sector may reflect multiple factors, including variance in employer hiring standards. Although studies comparing PSW education by sector indicate that PSWs working in the home and community have the lowest levels, within specific Canadian provinces, many such PSWs (up to 73 per cent) have reported educational attainment beyond high school (Zeytinoglu et al 2016). Immigrants employed as PSWs who previously worked as nurses in their home country may be contributing to the increased education levels reported in some samples. Aside from higher education levels, the appropriateness and applicability of education and training to PSW work is also an important consideration. Approximately 30 per cent of Canadian PSWs reported having no education related to their PSW position, with PSWs in long-term care the most likely to report that their education was closely related to their work (Zagrodney et al 2019).

An international scoping review (Hewko et al 2015) suggested that the number of years of PSW work experience ranged from 6.6 years in Japan (Nakanishi and Imai 2012) to 12.4 years in the United States (Castle et al 2007). PSWs with lower educational attainment and less experience generally earn lower wages (Price-Glynn and Rakovski 2012). On average, PSWs who did not graduate at high school earned 8.6 per cent less than those with high school diplomas, while PSWs with a bachelor's degree earned approximately 30 per cent more (Baughman and Smith 2008). Canadian PSWs working in the home and community with seven or more years of experience earned higher wages than those with less than seven years of experience (Home Care Sector Study Corporation 2003). Since education levels for the general Canadian population have also increased over time (Statistics Canada 2017) it is unclear whether more highly educated PSWs can necessarily expect to receive relatively higher wages in years to come.

Job characteristics and the relationship to labour market outcomes

Full-time, part-time, casual hours of work and job schedules

Although the PSW literature does not always distinguish between full-time hours and full-time positions, the number of full-time or FTE PSWs provides a more nuanced picture of supply than does the number of individuals employed. Some PSWs may work full-time hours without a full-time position (for example, part-time workers holding multiple part-time positions in different care settings), but full-time positions are usually associated with positive job features such as fringe benefits.

A scoping review of the international PSW literature (Hewko et al 2015) reported a wide range of PSWs holding full-time positions internationally and over an extended time period from 14.7 per cent in Canada (Bloom et al 2012) to 79.3 per cent in the United States. The 1993–2010 survey of Canadian PSWs placed them at the higher end of this range, with 63–70 per cent reporting full-time status across all sectors (Zagrodney et al 2019), although this was slightly lower than other health care occupations within Canada – including for RNs and LPNs (Pyper 2004). In addition, this study noted that Canadian PSWs had higher rates of temporary employment and were less likely to hold a permanent job compared to the nursing profession, reflecting the greater casual and transient nature of the PSW labour market than the nursing labour market. However, more recent national findings found that the majority (approximately 85 per cent) of Canadian PSWs did report having a permanent position (Zagrodney et al 2019).

In terms of sectoral discrepancies in Canada, hospital PSWs tend to have the highest rates of working full-time and the lowest rates of working on a casual basis (Department of Employment and Social Development Canada 2018), as well as the highest rates of full-year employment, permanent status, and the lowest number of unemployed or 'not in labour force' weeks (Montgomery et al 2005). PSWs in the home and community generally report the highest proportions working on a part-time or casual basis (Home Care Sector Study Corporation 2003; Montgomery et al 2005; Potter et al 2006; Sims-Gould et al 2010; Zeytinoglu et al 2014). They also have the highest proportions of working an irregular schedule or a split-shift (Zagrodney et al 2019) – and such irregular schedules are likely to negatively impact the ability of such PSWs to work more hours. Although individuals may prefer to work on a casual or part-time basis, previous studies suggest that many would prefer to work full time (Pyper 2004). Differences by sector exist here as well, where greater proportions of long-term care (21.6 per cent) and home and community (21.1 per cent) PSWs as opposed to hospital (9.1 per cent) PSWs wanted to work more hours (Zagrodney et al 2019).

The number of months that a PSW works for an employer is an indication of retention – a valued trait within a labour market anticipating a shortage of workers. The longer a PSW stays with a given employer, the more likely the PSW is to have acquired skills that are specific to that job and the more disruptive it may become for both employer and employee to switch to another job requiring different skills. The scoping review by Hewko and colleagues (2015) observed that the average job duration for PSWs ranged from 2.16 to 9.86 years. Another study found that Canadian PSWs were at the higher end of this spectrum, reporting an average job duration with a single employer of approximately 9 years. This differed by sector, with reported averages of 13 years for hospital PSWs, 9 years for long-term care, and 7 years for home and community (Zagrodney et al 2019).

Union status

Unions generally provide workers with a greater sense of unity, higher pay and job security (Long 1993). Such factors may influence retention and recruitment. Rates of union status for PSWs vary based on the specific sample. A scoping review found that approximately 10–19 per cent of PSWs were unionised (Hewko et al 2015). Past research indicates that home health care workers in Canada prefer work environments offering unionisation (Martin-Matthews et al 2011). However, for the Canadian PSW labour market, unionisation does not appear to guarantee wage or non-wage benefits such as insurance coverage. In a sample of PSWs where the majority were unionised (70 per cent), only half (51 per cent) received such benefits. In contrast, 80 per cent of nurses (both RNs and LPNs) were unionised, with 68 per cent of LPNs and 69 per cent of RNs receiving insurance coverage (Pyper 2004).

Union status for Canadian PSWs also varies by sector. Across a nationwide Canadian sample, unionisation was approximately 35 per cent in home and community, 68 per cent in long-term care, and 93 per cent in the hospital sector (Zagrodney et al 2019). PSWs working in home and community care with union status in Canada generally report higher wages than their non-unionised counterparts (Havens 2003; Home Care Sector Study Corporation 2003; Martin-Matthews and Sims-Gould 2008). However, the number of hours worked may also be affected, with some suggesting that unionisation can result in fewer hours worked due to enforced schedule restrictions (see, for example, Keefe et al 2011).

Benefits and pensions

Satisfaction with benefits may influence the decision of PSWs to remain in the PSW labour market. A review of the PSW literature shows that the scope of health insurance coverage for PSWs (which may include, for instance, full coverage for the individual or family coverage) varies significantly (Hewko et al 2015). Given that PSWs often experience high risk of injury on the job, health benefits are expected to be particularly important to this group. Yet research from the United States shows that female PSWs receive less coverage than women who work in non-PSW jobs (Baughman and Smith 2008; Potter et al 2006). Although in Canada, and many other jurisdictions in developed countries, PSWs are entitled to full public coverage for hospital and physician care, other costs (including rehabilitation and outpatient pharmaceuticals) may not be universally covered. Only one-quarter of a Canadian sample of PSWs were satisfied or very satisfied with the amount of benefits that they received (Zeytinoglu et al 2016). However, since greater benefits are more often offered for full-time employees, this may encourage PSWs to work full-time hours when the opportunity arises.

PSWs with lower wages also tend to receive lower benefits in the home and community sector in Canada (Keefe et al 2011). The relationship between wages and benefits is complex as many socio-demographic characteristics (for example, education) that affect wages are found to also affect whether PSWs are offered health insurance (Baughman and Smith 2008) and other benefits (Price-Glynn and Rakovski 2012). Sectoral discrepancies also exist, with PSWs working in hospitals being the most likely to receive benefits, followed by those in long-term care and home and community (Baughman and Smith 2008). Since pension amounts are typically decided based on total earnings (hours worked multiplied by hourly wage), expected pension income levels can also influence how long individuals remain in the labour market and how intensively (full-time, part-time or casual) a PSW is likely to work to accumulate pension benefits. Zagrodney and colleagues (2019) found that the likelihood of having a pension differs by sector and may influence an individual's sector choice as PSWs working in hospitals are most likely to receive a pension (80 per cent), followed by PSWs in the long-term care (50 per cent) and home and community (33 per cent) sectors. Improving job characteristics such as offering pension plans are therefore one avenue to consider if the aim is to improve retention and recruitment, especially within the home and community sector.

Conclusion

This chapter has offered a brief synopsis of the PSW labour market and highlighted important factors related to supply with this labour market, including differences by sector. The literature indicates multiple sectoral discrepancies among Canadian PSWs, in terms of both individual and socio-demographic characteristics and job characteristics which seem to be reflected in other jurisdictions. Sector-specific variations in such factors as gender, age, immigrant status, ethnicity, family and household characteristics, health, and education, and labour market outcomes of wages and hours have been noted. Job characteristics are also a vital component of supply within the labour market, where such factors as the number of permanent jobs on offer play a major role in securing and increasing PSW supply. The chapter also noted differences across sectors in labour supply outcomes and behaviours such as wages and hours worked, full-time, part-time, and casual hours of work, job schedules, unionisation, benefits and pensions. The heterogeneous nature of the PSW labour market is an important consideration in resource planning; sectoral differences are expected to impose differences on labour supply behaviours and outcomes.

Future directions in research relating to PSW supply in Canada and other international societies should look beyond the raw numbers of individuals and FTEs that will be required to meet rising demands and include analysis of the appropriateness of workers (in terms of factors such as education and training) to meet specific and evolving patient needs. The role that registries and other regulatory practices play in terms of the monitoring and managing the supply of PSWs should be considered, along with the impact that such processes may have on supply. Enforcement of any future or current regulations and potential impacts on the labour market are crucial given the expected gap between supply and demand for PSWs. Future research could then provide evidence on the impact of such policy shifts and/or regulations on labour market outcomes for PSWs. In filling this gap, a possible broadening of recruitment strategies beyond groups currently working as PSWs – who are largely a female, older workforce – may be helpful. Given the increasing role of PSWs in Canada as well as in many other countries internationally, such future work would be of high value; there are real possibilities here of utilising such information to learn from each other and inform PSW-related initiatives on a global scale.

References

Alamgir, H., Cvitkovich, Y., Yu, S. and Yassi, A. (2007) 'Work-related injury among direct care occupations in British Columbia, Canada', *Occupational and Environmental Medicine* 64(11): 769–75.

Alamgir, H., Yu, S., Chavoshi, N. and Ngan, K. (2008) 'Occupational injury among full-time, part-time and casual health care workers', *Occupational Medicine* 58(5): 348–54.

Aoki, M. (2016) 'Nursing care workers hard to find but in demand in aging Japan', *Japan Times* 27 June.

Baughman, R. and Smith, K. (2008) 'Employment transitions of direct care workers: Where do they go and why?', Conference on Health, Health Insurance and Labor Markets, 3 October, http://citeseerx.ist.psu.edu/viewdoc/download?doi=10.1.1.187.2210&rep=rep1&type=pdf

Baughman, R. and Smith, K. (2012) 'Labor mobility of the direct care workforce: implications for the provision of long-term care', *Health Economics* 21(12): 1402–15.

Behan, J., Condon, N., Milicevic, I., Shally, C. and Saothair, I.F.A. (2009) 'A quantitative tool for workforce planning in healthcare: example simulations', Dublin: Skills and Labour Market Research Unit on behalf of the Expert Group on Future Skills Needs, www.skillsireland.ie/media/egfsn090617_healthcare_report.pdf

Berta, W., Laporte, A., Deber, R., Baumann, A. and Gamble, B. (2013) 'The evolving role of health care aides in the long-term care and home and community care sectors in Canada', *Human Resources for Health* 11(25).

Bloom, J., Duckett, S. and Robertson, A. (2012) 'Development of an interactive model for planning the care workforce for Alberta: Case study', *Human Resources for Health* 10(22).

Bureau of Labor Statistics (2015) 'Nursing assistants and orderlies', Washington DC: US Department of Labor, www.bls.gov/ooh/healthcare/nursing-assistants.htm

Canadian Home Care Association (2008) 'Portraits of home care in Canada', Ottawa: Canadian Home Care Association.

Canadian Occupational Projection System (2017a) 'Occupation data, occupational projection summary: Home support workers, housekeepers and related occupations (4412)', Ottawa: Government of Canada, http://occupations.esdc.gc.ca/sppc-cops/occupationsummarydetail.jsp?&tid=150

Canadian Occupational Projection System (2017b) 'Occupation data, occupational projection summary: Nurse aides, orderlies and patient service associates and other assisting occupations in support of health services (3413)', Ottawa: Government of Canada, http://occupations.esdc.gc.ca/sppc-cops/occupationsummarydetail.jsp?&tid=150

Carstairs, S. and Keon, W.J. (2007) *Special Senate Committee on Aging. First Interim Report: Embracing the Challenge of Aging*, Ottawa: Senate of Canada, March, https://sencanada.ca/content/sen/Committee/391/agei/rep/repintfeb07-e.pdf

Castle, N.G., Engberg, J., Anderson, R. and Men, A. (2007) 'Job satisfaction of nurse aides in nursing homes: Intent to leave and turnover', *The Gerontologist* 47(2): 193–204.

Deber, R. (2018) *Treating Health Care: How the Canadian System Works and How It Could Work Better*, Toronto: University of Toronto Press.

Denton, M., Zeytinoglu, I.U., Davies, S. and Hunter, D. (2006) 'The impact of implementing managed competition on home care workers' turnover decisions', *Healthcare Policy* 1(4): 106–23.

Department of Employment and Social Development Canada (2017a) 'Personal support aide – medical in Canada: Job market report wages', Ottawa: Government of Canada, www.jobbank.gc.ca/marketreport/wages-occupation/15789/ca

Department of Employment and Social Development Canada (2017b) 'Personal support worker – home support in Canada: Job market report wages', Ottawa: Government of Canada, www.jobbank.gc.ca/marketreport/wages-occupation/24584/ca

Department of Employment and Social Development Canada (2018) 'Personal support worker – home support in Canada: Job market report outlook', Ottawa: Government of Canada, www.jobbank.gc.ca/marketreport/outlook-occupation/24584/ca

Dill, D.M., Keefe, J.M. and McGrath, D.S. (2012) 'The influence of intrinsic and extrinsic job values on turnover intention among continuing care assistants in Nova Scotia', *Home Health Care Services Quarterly* 31(2): 111–29.

Foerster, V. and Murtagh, J. (2013) 'British Columbia care aide and community health worker registry: A review', British Columbia: Ministry of Health, www.health.gov.bc.ca/library/publications/year/2013/bc-care-aide-registry-report.pdf

Fujisawa, R. and Colombo, F. (2009) 'The long-term care workforce: overview and strategies to adapt supply to a growing demand', *OECD Health Working Papers 44*, http://envejecimiento.csic.es/documentos/documentos/fujisawa-longterm-01.pdf

Government of Quebec (2016) 'Préposé ou préposée d'aide à domicile', Emploi-Québec, Government of Quebec, www.emploiquebec.gouv. qc.ca/citoyens/developper-et-faire-reconnaitre-vos-competences/ qualification-professionnelle/qualification-volontaire/liste-des-metiers/prepose-ou-preposee-daide-a-domicile/

Hamadi, H., Probst, J.C., Khan, M.M., Bellinger, J. and Porter, C. (2016) 'Home-based direct care workers: Their reported injuries and perceived training knowledge', *Workplace Health and Safety* 64(6): 249–61.

Havens, B. (2003) 'Canadian home care human resources study-synthesis report', Ottawa: The Home Care Sector Study Corporation.

Health Council of Canada (2012) *Seniors in Need, Caregivers in Distress: What Are the Home Care Priorities for Seniors?* Ottawa: HCC.

Health Professions Regulatory Advisory Council (2006) 'The regulation of personal support workers', Toronto: HPRAC.

Hegewisch, A. and Liepmann, H. (2010) 'Fact sheet: the gender wage gap by occupation', *Institute for Women's Policy Research*, Washington DC: IWPR.

Hewko, S.J., Cooper, S.L., Huynh, H., Spiwek, T.L., Carleton, H.L., Reid, S. and Cummings, G.G. (2015) 'Invisible no more: A scoping review of the health care aide workforce literature', *BMC Nursing* 14(38).

Home Care Sector Study Corporation (2003) 'Canadian home care human resources study', Ottawa: CHWN.

Keefe, J.M., Knight, L., Martin-Matthews, A. and Legare, J. (2011) 'Key issues in human resource planning for home support workers in Canada', *Work* 40(1): 21–8.

Korczyk, S.M. (2004) 'Long-term workers in five countries: Issues and options', *American Association of Retired Persons Public Policy Institute*, Washington DC: AARP.

Long, R.J. (1993) 'The effect of unionization on employment growth of Canadian companies', *Industrial and Labour Relations Review* 46(4): 691–703.

Lum, J.M., Sladek, J. and Ying, A. (2015) 'Ontario personal support workers in home and community care: CRNCC/PSNO survey results', *Canadian Research Network for Care in the Community*, Toronto: CRNCC.

Martin-Matthews, A. and Sims-Gould, J. (2008) 'Employers, home support workers and elderly clients: Identifying key issues in delivery and receipt of home support', *Healthcare Quarterly* 11(4): 69–75.

Martin-Matthews, A., Sims-Gould, J. and Naslund, J. (2011) 'Ethno-cultural diversity in home care work in Canada: Issues confronted, strategies employed', *International Journal of Ageing and Later Life* 5(2): 77–101.

Ministry of Health and Long-term Care (2015) 'Ontario increasing wages for personal support workers: province continuing to invest in home and community care', Toronto: Queen's Printer for Ontario, 22 June, www.health.gov.on.ca/en/news/bulletin/2015/hb_20150622.aspx

Minister of Health Seniors and Active Living. (2016) 'Future of home care services in Manitoba', Government of Manitoba, www.gov.mb.ca/health/homecare/future_homecare.pdf

Montgomery, R.J.V., Holley, L., Deichert, J. and Kosloski, K. (2005) 'A profile of home care workers from the 2000 census: How it changes what we know', *The Gerontologist* 45(5): 593–600.

Nakanishi, M. and Imai, H. (2012) 'Job role quality and intention to leave current facility and to leave profession of direct care workers in Japanese residential facilities for elderly', *Archives of Gerontology and Geriatrics* 54(1): 102–108.

National Nursing Assessment Service (2018) 'RN, RPN, and LPN requirements in Canada', www.nnas.ca/nursing-requirements-in-canada/

Potter, S.J., Churilla, A. and Smith, K. (2006) 'An examination of full-time employment in the direct-care workforce', *Journal of Applied Gerontology* 25(5): 356–74.

Price-Glynn, K. and Rakovski, C. (2012) 'Who rides the glass escalator? Gender, race and nationality in the national nursing assistant study', *Work, Employment and Society* 26(5): 699–715.

Pyper, W. (2004) 'Employment trends in nursing', cat. no. 75-001-XIE, Statistics Canada, www150.statcan.gc.ca/n1/en/pub/75-001-x/11104/7611-eng.pdf?st=JZLoEaDJ

Rhéaume, A., Dykeman, M., Davidson, P. and Ericson, P. (2007) 'The impact of health care restructuring and baccalaureate entry to practice on nurses in New Brunswick', *Policy, Politics and Nursing Practice* 8(2): 130–39.

Roberts, K., Rao, D., Bennett, T., Loukine, L. and Jayaraman, G. (2015) 'Prevalence and patterns of chronic disease multimorbidity and associated determinants in Canada', *Health Promotion and Chronic Disease Prevention in Canada: Research, Policy and Practice* 35(6): 87–94.

Saks, M. (2010) 'Analyzing the professions: The case for the neo-Weberian approach', *Comparative Sociology* 9(6): 887–915.

Sims-Gould, J., Byrne, K., Craven, C., Martin-Matthews, A. and Keefe, J. (2010) 'Why I became a home support worker: Recruitment in the home health sector', *Home Health Care Services Quarterly* 29(4): 171–94.

Statistics Canada (1996) '1996 census of population: Electronic area profiles', October.

Statistics Canada (2006) 'Aboriginal identity population by age groups, median age and sex, percentage distribution for both sexes, for Canada, provinces and territories – 20% sample data'.

Statistics Canada (2016) '2016 census of population: Electronic area profiles', November.

Statistics Canada (2017) 'Education in Canada: Key results from the 2016 census', Statistics Canada: The Daily, November.

Tijdens, K., De Vries, D.H. and Steinmetz, S. (2013) 'Health workforce remuneration: Comparing wage levels, ranking, and dispersion of 16 occupational groups in 20 countries', *Human Resources for Health* 11(11).

Weber, M. (1968) *Economy and Society: An Outline of Interpretive Sociology*, New York: Bedminster Press.

Zagrodney, K., Deber, R., Saks, M. and Laporte, A. (2019) 'Differences in PSW job characteristics and labour supply behaviours by care sector: The disadvantaged home and community PSW', Global Carework Summit, Toronto, June.

Zarnett, D., Coyte, P.C., Nauenberg, E., Doran, D. and Laporte, A. (2009) 'The effects of competition on community-based nursing wages', *Healthcare Policy* 4(3): e129–44.

Zelisko, D., Baumann, A., Gamble, B., Laporte, A. and Deber, R. (2014) 'Ensuring accountability through health professional regulatory bodies: The case of conflict of interest', *Healthcare Policy* 10(SP): 110–20.

Zeytinoglu, I., Brookman, C., Denton, M., VanderBent, S., Boucher, P. and Davies, S. (2016) 'The PSW health and safety matters survey: PSWs have a say – What we heard about training and injuries at work: Survey results', *Ontario Community Support Association Webinar*, June, Toronto: OCSA, www.pswshaveasay.ca/survey-results.html

Zeytinoglu, I.U., Denton, M., Brookman, C. and Plenderleith, J. (2014) 'Task shifting policy in Ontario, Canada: Does it help personal support workers' intention to stay?', *Health Policy* 117(2): 179–86.

ELEVEN

The role of health support workers in the ageing crisis

Miwako Hosoda

Introduction: Care work in an ageing society

Peterson (1999:43) wrote over 20 years ago that: 'Aging has become a truly global challenge and must therefore be given high priority on the global policy agenda'. Today, the world, in both developed and developing countries, is ageing (Shetty 2012). When the World Health Assembly was held in May 2016, 194 countries expressed the idea that every country should have a long-term care system. Although there are still few countries that have such a system, care services for elderly people are operated under various systems by each of these countries (World Health Organization 2019). In Japan, the Long-Term Care Insurance System (LTCIS) was introduced in 2000. Under the System, care services by qualified workers, such as Certified Care Workers (CCWs) and Home Visiting Care Workers (HVCWs), are covered by insurance. Despite the implementation of the system, there are some problems and challenges associated with these and other workers in this sector, as will be explored in this chapter after first setting a context.

The response to ageing in Japan

While the ageing population is growing globally, Japan in particular can be described as a super ageing society. It is expected that one-third of the population will be over 65 years old, and one of the fifth will be over 75 years in 2025 (National Institute of Population and Social Security Research 2017). There is also a tendency for single or married people to live apart from other family members, when incidences of elderly dementia are increasing. Concerns over such circumstances have been expressed since the 1990s, and different ways of caring for the elderly have been sought. Traditionally, families have taken care of the elderly, but currently family care is considered to be difficult. For example, Zarit and colleagues (1986:261) wrote that 'caregivers perceived their emotional or physical health, social life, and financial status as suffering as a result of caring for their relatives'. The family's shape has also changed – from the extended family to the nuclear family – and care provided outside the family is now a requirement. In the past elderly care was provided within the framework of the Medical Insurance System (MIS), which led to an increase in medical costs. The MIS covers medical treatment due to illness, injury, preparation for hospitalisation, surgery, outpatient visits and medication. But this has resulted in rapidly escalating medical expenses in Japan. In response to these phenomena – especially the call for care providers other than family members to be involved and for elderly care separate from insured medical care – the LTCIS was introduced from 2000 by the Ministry of Health, Labor and Welfare (MHLW) to make elderly care sustainable in the future.

Medical and nursing care systems supporting the elderly

In Japan all citizens had to subscribe to the MIS that started in 1961 and to the LTCIS that supplanted it from 2000. Under the LTCIS, everyone over the age of 45 has to pay fees to insurers through local municipalities. When a person reaches the age of over 65 years old (45 years old in the case of a disability) and needs care, this individual (or a family member) must submit an application for care services to the insurers. The insurers then approve or otherwise a certain amount of care according to the needs of the insured. These are determined by the certification committee for long-term care, who are mostly members of the medical profession. Thereafter the insured requests a care manager to create a personalised care plan. Following this, the care manager introduces the insured to the relevant care service providers. According to the care plan, care workers with certain qualifications belonging to the care service provider deliver the service. When insured people receive a care service, they pay 10 per cent of the cost. The remaining 90 per cent of the cost is paid by the municipal insurer to the care service provider. According to the census conducted by the MHLW (2017), there are almost 34 million primary insured people, and 6 million individuals use the care service provided by the LTCIS each year. The scheme covers home services such as home visits, nursing, short-stay admissions and long-term care support. This is in addition to services including outpatient day care and rehabilitation, residential care for conditions like dementia, and community provision based on multifunctional long-term care in small group homes, and communal daily care.

The professional involvement of doctors and nurses in the Long-term Care Insurance Scheme

Professionals involved in providing such care services include doctors, nurses, care managers, care support specialists, CCWs and HVCWs. The care manager has an additional certificate, which doctors, dentists, pharmacists, public health nurses, nurses, nutritionists, physiotherapists, occupational therapists, social workers and care workers are eligible to obtain. Doctors, nurses and care managers are responsible for creating care plans and giving advice on what facilities and types of care are suitable for the elderly who are in need. According to the care plan, CCWs provide services for the elderly. From a neo-Weberian point of view, medical dominance is well known in the health field (Saks 2016) and is also replicated in the care field in relationships with nurses and other care workers in Japan. According to the Japan Medical Association (JMA), the largest medical association in Japan, the role of doctors in the LTCIS is to maintain and improve the quality of life of the elderly. This lead role is based on their full exclusionary social closure in neo-Weberian terms (Saks 2010). The JMA (1999) introduced three types of duties in this respect for medical doctors:

• Consultation and advice giving for local residents, including both the elderly and their families.
• Providing information and instruction for home service companies and home care support companies making care plans for the elderly.
• Providing medical services in institutions and at the homes of the elderly.

While the client is using home and other services such as visiting nursing care, doctors act as leaders who review the care plan through continuous medical management, including hospitalisation and admission, choice of the type of home care and/or institutional facilities. Medical doctors are also importantly expected to determine an individual's level of care needs. There are seven levels of care needs, related to the amount of care covered by LTCIS. Medical doctors give advice to care managers and review the degree of care from time to time (JMA 1999). Doctors therefore not only had a dominant role in the medical field under the MIS, but also in the care practice field under the LTCIS.

The Japan Nursing Association (JNA), with which most nurses, midwives, and public health nurses are registered, also defines the role of nurses in the care field as leaders. According to the JNA (2016):

- Nurses should do regular nursing work at medical facilities and the residence of the elderly and make medical judgements which care workers are not allowed to do.
- Nurses are expected to provide medical care for the elderly in cooperation with doctors and other care workers.
- Nurses are expected to provide care not only for the elderly, but also their family members (including mental support), and to facilitate their decision making.

Furthermore, according to the JNA, the power of nurses in the medical field is large, but when nurses work in the care field, they are in a higher position than care workers. Therefore, there is a hierarchy in the care field. Certified and uncertified care workers work in care. More qualified care workers include CCWs and HVCWs who used to be called home helpers and uncertified care workers. The hierarchy is observed at each level of care work. Thus, there are boundary issues in providing care services among doctors, nurses and care workers, which will be explored later in this chapter. However, doctors' and nurses' power seems less strong in the care field than in the medical and health field because it mainly involves making care plans, with decision making in practice undertaken by individual care workers.

The Certified Care Worker and Home Visiting Care Worker

CCWs and HVCWs have responsibility for providing care services under the LTCIS. A CCW is the only nationally qualified health care worker specialising in nursing care. The HVCW is based on undergoing training approved by prefectural governors and operated by private training institutes and local government. Insured elderly users receive a care service from CCWs and HVCWs through the LTCIS. We shall now discuss the role of each of these higher level support workers in turn.

Certified Care Workers

A CCW is based on a national qualification under the 1987 Social Worker and Certified Care Worker Act. The work of the CCW is to provide a care service according to the needs of the person by responding to the care plan. As such, the CCW supports the daily life of elderly people and those with disabilities. The CCW sometimes also provides guidance on nursing care for lay caregivers such as families and volunteers.

There are two main ways to acquire a CCW qualification. First, aspirants can graduate from the training facility designated by the MHLW, such as junior colleges and vocational schools, and then study for two years (1,850 hours) to take the CCW national examination. Second, those who have engaged in work such as nursing care for three years or more can simply take the CCW national examination. Many of those with CCW certificates have more than three years' work experience in nursing care and have passed the CCW examination.

The work of a CCW varies widely. For example, it may include personal assistance for elderly people and those with a disability to move, eat, bathe, keep clean and sleep. In addition, health maintenance, housekeeping assistance, nursing care, cooperation with other occupations, and counselling may also be included in the role. However, CCWs cannot conduct medical practice. Nonetheless, with the revision of the 2011 Social Worker and Care Workers Law, medical practices, such as sputum suction and tube nutrition, were added to the work of CCWs. It thereafter became possible for them to perform at least some part of what had previously been regarded as exclusively medical practice. The place of work of CCWs can vary – ranging from special nursing homes for the elderly and nursing home health care facilities to day service centres, group homes and people's own homes. More than 90 per cent of CCWs are women. The number is increasing every year and, as of 2016, there are nearly 1.5 million people who fulfil this role (MHLW 2016). Some 60 per cent of CCWs are in their 40s and 50s. The average salary is about 300,000 yen per month, which is lower than a nurse's salary of 400,000 yen.

Home Visiting Care Workers

HVCWs provide a visiting care service based on the LTCIS, after they have completed the prescribed training. In the past home helpers had training courses at first-grade and second-grade level, but they were abolished and unified as a result of the revision of the qualification system in 2013. HVCW training is provided by private training institutions and local government, as designated by prefectural governors. A certificate of completion is issued after an HVCW has taken a 130-hour training course and passed an examination. The job of an HVCW is to visit the residences of elderly people and disabled people who need care and to support their daily living so that they can live independently in their local community.

The care services of HVCWs are determined by the LTCIS Law and include body care services and daily living assistance. Body care services incorporate, among other things, helping with meals, bathing, excretion, posture enhancement and hospital visits. Life support services such as cooking, washing, receiving medicine and shopping are also carried out by the HVCW, in consultation with family members. A daily living assistance service is provided as well in a range of areas from spiritual care to giving supplementary support in the transition from home to hospital. The workplace of the HVCW is where the person who needs nursing care lives or a dedicated apartment/house for the elderly, with a nursing care service. Currently, the number of HVCWs is over 460,000 and nearly 70 per cent of employment is part time, in a situation where 90 per cent of staff are female. The average age of a HVCW is 52.7 years old. Over half are aged 40 and above. About 30 per cent of HVCWs are over 60 years old. The average monthly salary is about 200,000 yen (MHLW 2013).

The differences between Certified Care Workers and Home Visit Care Workers

The jobs of CCWs and HVCWs are basically the same. However, CCWs hold national qualifications, and can be responsible persons at nursing homes and provide nursing care guidance to other caregivers. In addition, a nursing care facility with a CCW receives extra payment from municipalities under certain conditions. There are also differences between CCWs and HVCWs in terms of both employment and treatment. The CCW can apply to a wider range of employers and is employed as a full-time worker by care service facilities and providers. The HVCW is most often employed on a part-time basis. Even though the CCW and HVCW do similar work, the CCW earns more due to the higher-level qualification obtained.

The less qualified health support worker: the *Tsukisoifu*

CCWs and HVCWs operate under the LTCIS; these are formal care service jobs in the social system. However, in order to support the daily lives of elderly people, the services received under the LTCIS are insufficient. Who provides the care not covered by the LTCIS? Here the *Tsukisoifu* or lower level support worker is a key care provider.

Brief history

The *Tsukisoifu* are women who used to stay with a patient in hospital, taking care of them and keeping the environment clean. *Tsukisoi* means attendant, and *fu* means woman. Originally in Japan before the Second World War, many hospitals and clinics were operated by doctors, and general nursing care and personal care of hospitalised patients were considered to be outside medical treatment (Sugiyama 1995). Care work for sick people was therefore undertaken by families and the *Tsukisoifu*. They brought a stove and pot into the hospital room to prepare meals and made up their bed next to the sick person to stay day and night (Hosoda 2012). Traditionally, the Japanese have a culture that thinks of someone in the family accompanying a hospitalised patient in this way is a virtue. As a Japanese social norm, there was a strong belief that, when a family member was hospitalised, the rest of the family should attend and care.

However, in modern hospitals, nursing care is included in medical treatment. From 1950 a 'complete nursing system' was implemented, and the *Tsukisoifu* were not admitted to care for family members. Nevertheless, the number of nurses was still insufficient, and it was increasingly felt that the care of the patient could not be realised without family and the *Tsukisoifu*. Therefore, care by family members and the *Tsukisoifu* continued. According to a survey by the JNA in 1980, there was some such person to care for the sick person at 88.3 per cent of 2,464 hospitals, and 11.2 per cent of these were *Tsukisoifu*. In the comparative survey by the JNA in 1991, there were such caregivers in 23.8 per cent of local hospitals, of whom 41.9 per cent were family members and 58.1 per cent were *Tsukisoifu* (JNA 1993).

Following on from this, a 'standardised nursing system' to secure a certain number of nurses in the hospital eventually began to be developed, and caregivers in hospital, including family members and the *Tsukisoifu*, were abolished in 1996. At this point there were 110,000 *Tsukisoifu*. This large job loss was a major social problem, and concerns arose about the shortage of nursing care for hospitalised patients. This issue featured in a television programme by the Japan Broadcast Association (NHK: *Nihon Hoso Kyokai*). Although the *Tsukisoifu* disappeared from hospitals, nursing care at home was necessary afterwards. A place where the *Tsukisoifu* could work therefore continued to be provided. Furthermore, in recent years, government policy in elderly care has been shifted from institutions to the home. As a consequence, demand for *Tsukisoifu* is growing, although the fees for the *Tsukisoifu* as a lower level support worker are not covered by LTCIS and users pay the full cost themselves.

I shall now describe what a *Tsukisoifu* does in more detail based on an interview with a *Tsukisoifu*, Ms A. Before starting the interview with Ms A, I explained to her the main purpose of the survey – namely, to examine the actual role and situation of a *Tsukisoifu* and to keep the interview anonymous. I told Ms A that cooperation in this interview was voluntary and oral consent for conducting the interview was given. In addition, I used materials in my research such as *Looking at a Number of Deaths* (Arai 1991), which was written about the experiences of the *Tsukisoifu*, and the websites of *Tsukisoifu* recruiting agencies.

The narratives of a Tsukisoifu

The actual condition of the *Tsukisoifu* has not been much studied. Even their numbers are not accurately known. There are several reasons for this, but the primary reason is that the *Tsukisoifu* herself does not positively grasp her existence. As Arai (1991: 20) says in her book, based on her own experiences as a *Tsukisoifu*: 'A *Tsukisoifu* [is] … a withered woman living at the bottom of society.' It was difficult to get acquainted with a *Tsukisoifu* who thought herself to be at the base of society. It was a rare opportunity to hear the story of a *Tsukisoifu* in a research interview. Ms A was 77 years old and had divorced in her thirties, and started to work as a *Tsukisoifu* to raise her children as a single mother. Her experiences as a *Tsukisoifu* had already covered nearly 40 years of work. In response to the question of why she continued to work in this role, she said:

> 'I do not get an answer, I was thinking I would have stopped this job after working 5 years, but I continued to work … [and] just bullied my body.' (Interview with Ms A, 13 November 2018)

Ms A has been working as a *Tsukisoifu* and home helper since the 1980s. She registered with a recruitment agency, having been introduced to her work through this agency. In 1988 she took a nursing assistant course which was sponsored by the agency and obtained a certificate. On the course, among other things, she learned about changing nappies, posture enhancement, and how to help the elderly sit on a chair. And in 1999 just before the LTCIS began, she took a second-grade course on the Tokyo home helper training programme and received a certificate of completion. The home helper was later called a HVCW. At the moment, Ms A was working sometimes as a *Tsukisoifu* and sometimes as a home helper.

Normally Ms A worked for one elderly person who was living at their own home in the community. But she was sometimes asked by a recruiting agency to go to another elderly person at the same time. From 2008 to 2018, Ms A regularly visited Ms B's house twice, sometimes three times, each week. Ms B was in her late 80s. Sometimes Ms A stayed overnight at Ms B's house and provided nursing care. Ms A's work was cooking, cleaning up after meals, room cleaning, washing and ironing. Besides the caring work for Ms B, Ms A sometimes washed and ironed for Ms B's family members.

As previously noted, for elderly people who need care to live in the community, the services covered by LTCIS are not enough. Furthermore, since Ms B's family also worked, they needed help with the household chores, in addition to nursing care. Therefore in order to provide necessary services for the elderly and their family, Ms A worked as a HVCW, *Tsukisoifu* and housekeeper, and provided comprehensive services for the family.

Table 11.1 shows the typical schedule for Ms A as a *Tsukisoifu/* housekeeper and a HVCW for a week at Ms B's home. When there was a request, and when it was possible temporally and physically, Ms A worked for other elderly people to provide care. At Ms B's house, when Ms A did not come, the family members took turns to take time off work and care for Ms B.

Ms A is a part-time worker and her salary is paid hourly. According to her, the hourly wage was 1,200 yen (about 10 Euros) when she worked as a housekeeper, and from 1,800 to 2,000 yen when she worked as a *Tsukisoifu*. She remembered that she earned 32,000 yen for a day of care (including an overnight stay). Ms A said: 'The wage seems fine, but I have to work all day and night, so I can work only two or three days a week'. She received additional transportation expenses, but even if she gave long-term care and stayed overnight, she had to pay for her own meals.

When I interviewed Ms A, it was just after Ms B who had been in care for ten years passed away. The first time Ms A met Ms B, the latter

Table 11.1: Ms A's weekly schedule (from the interview, November 2018)

Mon	
Tue	
Wed	9:00–17:00 Worked as *Tsukisoifu/*housekeeper. Sometimes stayed overnight.
Thu	9:00–17:00 Worked as *Tsukisoifu/*housekeeper. 17:00–19:00 Worked as HVCW.
Fri	
Sat	9:00–20:00 Worked as *Tsukisoifu/*housekeeper. Sometimes stayed overnight.
Sun	

had just returned from hospital to her own home. She was hospitalised due to a stroke (cerebral infarction) and had a gastric fistula on her stomach. Ms A thought that it would be nice for Ms B to be able to eat using her mouth. So Ms A cooked a meal which Ms B liked and chopped it into small pieces at home, packed it in a container, and brought it to Ms B's home. Then Ms A tried to make Ms B eat a meal little by little. Ms A voluntarily made a meal at her home for Ms B, but did not receive any fee for making meals. Yet Ms A continued to do it. After a year of repeating these things, Ms B finally could eat from her mouth. A gastric fistula was no longer necessary. Ms A was praised by Ms B's home physician for this achievement. Ms A said she was so happy and proud of herself at that time.

Still, Ms A said that the work of the *Tsukisoifu* is 'worthless'. And, she added 'I'm thinking of stopping this work because Ms B passed away', noting that:

> 'I am overwhelmed to work as a *Tsukisoifu*. In addition to the care of patients, I have also done laundry, cleaning, ironing, preparing meals, cleaning-up for the whole family.' (Interview with Ms A, 13 November 2018)

The work of the *Tsukisoifu* therefore seems to have no breaks and boundaries in time and emotional feeling. Comprehensive care for the elderly is carried out by the devotion and sacrifice of the *Tsukisoifu*. But the sustainability of the elderly home care system can be doubted as it is and a solution needs to be found.

How the work of the lower level support workers operates

Many of the *Tsukisoifu* are registered at employment agencies and receive work from agent referrals. The agencies are licensed by the MHLW based on the Employment Security Law. Once the *Tsukisoifu* is introduced to a user by the agent, the *Tsukisoifu* provides a nursing care service which is not covered by the LTCIS. Since the cost of a *Tsukisoifu* is not covered by insurance, the users pay the full expenses themselves and also pay a referral fee to the agency.

The *Tsukisoifu*'s work is diverse as a lower level support worker – it may involve care ranging from toiletry to dietary assistance. The *Tsukisoifu*'s work also includes household chores in general, such as laundry, wiping windows, drying futons, replacing light bulbs, garbage disposal and weeding in the garden. The *Tsukisoifu* accompanies elderly persons when they go shopping, to the bank, to the post office, for a walk and other outings. The *Tsukisoifu's* salary is paid hourly or daily. According to the website of an agency, the average wage is about 1,000 yen to 1,500 yen per hour. In the case of staying overnight, it is about 10,000 yen a day (for 11 hours actual working time).

Boundary issues in care

The role of higher level support workers, such as CCWs and HVCWs, and the lowlier *Tsukisoifu* in medical and nursing care workplaces has been reviewed in this chapter. The *Tsukisoifu* are being forgotten by society, although the necessity of their role has not diminished. The importance of care services for the elderly is increasing, but there are several challenges posed by the care services given by these caregivers. These are common not only to *Tsukisoifu* and housekeepers, who are not required to obtain qualifications, but also to CCWs and HVCWs who have certifications and qualifications. In this regard, there are particular problems surrounding the boundaries of care work in the hierarchy of medical and nursing professionals and care workers. These relate to issues based on the distinction between medical care and nursing care, between nursing care and living assistance in daily life, and between paid care and family care in Japanese society, which have ambiguous boundaries. In addition, the paid caring and support occupations at the bottom of the hierarchy appear unstable and have the mark of precarity. These issues will now be examined.

Between medical care and other forms of care

The boundary between medical and other forms of care is ambiguous. This problem is not only faced by *Tsukisoifu,* but also other care workers like the CCWs and HVCWs. According to the Medical Practitioners' Act, the Dentist's Act, and the Public Health Nurses, Midwives and Nurses Act, providing medical care is prohibited for those who do not have licences. For example, an HVCW injecting insulin into a care recipient breaks the law. If you are a diabetic, you can inject insulin by yourself. But those who can provide insulin injections are formally limited to doctors and nurses. However, care workers actually often carry out such tasks in their workplaces (Shinozaki 2002). 'Stool extraction', 'treatment of bedsores' and 'medication management' are also exclusive medical activities, but these too are frequently carried out in practice by care workers on site.

When a user is constipated, a care worker may provide a glycerin enema or a stool excretion. Traditionally, caregivers were not allowed to carry out glycerin enemas, but in 2005 the Director of the Medical Division of the MHLW issued medical notice 0726005 and disposable glycerin enemas can now beprovided by care workers. However, although this accentuates the ambiguity of roles, stool excretion is still designated as a fee-based medical practice as there is a danger of damaging or perforating the rectal wall if the stool excretion is carried out without experience or preparation. There are also risks of haemoglobinuria and haemolysis if patients have rectal diseases such as haemorrhoids and rectal cancer. Some elderly patients, who have blood pressure fluctuations due to general conditions such as heart disease, may also be adversely affected by invasive stool extraction. With many adverse events reported (see, for instance, Akeno et al 2017), there are arguments for restricting such procedures to doctors and registered nurses (Ohnishi and Ohnishi 2009; Shiraishi 2013). Even so, care workers still carry out illegal procedures in practice to respond to the needs of the elderly, with all the associated risks involved (Okamoto et al 2006; Sasaki and Takiuchi 2009; Shinozaki 2008).

There are also many other operations that are at the boundary between medical care and other forms of care. One survey asked HVCWs and other care staff which medical care they had carried out within the past year from the list shown in Table 11.2 (Shinozaki 2005). Of 216 respondents, 38 (17.6 per cent) answered 'I always did one of those', 177 respondents (81.9 per cent) answered 'I sometimes did one of those'. So, 99.5 per cent of nursing and care workers had used some form of medical care.

Whether such an act is an abuse of medical practice is partly based on the physical condition of the patient/user and how the action is performed. The 2005 announcement from the Director of MHLW,

Table 11.2: Items mentioned as medical practice

Applying a poultice	Applying ointment
Administering eye drops	Cutting rolled and ringworm nails
Changing bedsore dressings	Suppository
Assessing blood pressure	Enema
Stool excretion	Suction of sputum
Preparation and management of oxygen inhalation	Removing intravenous needles
Management of abnormal anus	Insulin injection
Withdrawing urine	Putting medicine directly in the user's mouth

though, indicated the care services which are not medical care and allowed care workers without a medical professional licence to operate on their own in certain circumstances. According to this announcement, interventions that are not considered to be medical practices include, among other things, measuring body temperature with a thermometer, measuring blood pressure with an automatic blood pressure device, treatments requiring no special judgement or technique for minor scratches and burns (including the replacement of dirty gauze), cutting nails, oral care, and extracting earwax. Nonetheless, sputum suction and tube feeding have for long been considered as medical practice and only doctors and nurses have been allowed to perform them according to the law. However, even here voices calling for a revocation led to part of the Certified Social Worker and Certified Care Worker Act being revised – and care workers with certain training became able to perform sputum suction under the authority of doctors and nurses from 2012 onwards (MHLW 2018a). This demonstrates that the boundaries between care workers and doctors and nurses are more fluid than meets the eye and may be mediated – as accentuated by neo-Weberian analysis – by power and interests, as well as public benefit (Saks 2016).

Between care and life support

We shall now look at the boundary between official care and daily life support. Daily life support covered by LTCIS varies, but is still limited for elderly people who live alone in the community. If elderly people live with their family, they cannot receive a daily living assistance service covered by LTCIS. Therefore, services exceeding the range of daily life, such as large-scale cleaning, rearrangement of furniture, pruning of plants and cooking for special occasions, like the New Year's Day Festival, cannot be covered. However, even if families live together, elderly households may need daily living assistance. They otherwise have to ask for such things as opening and closing curtains, replacing bulbs, changing the arrangement of the room and preparing meals (Mizuho Information and Research Institute 2012) – services that are difficult to provide under the LTCIS. In addition, the time range for receiving services each day is also limited. *Tsukisoifu* and housekeepers will therefore typically be responsible for such services. As described, Ms A cooked a special meal for Ms B at her own home, and packed this in a container and carried it to Ms B's house. Ms A preferred to use her own kitchen and did not have enough time to cook while she was doing care work at Ms B's house. As Ms A said:

'I wanted to do this for Ms B. as much as I can. However, I could not know which job is as a HVCW, a *Tsukisoifu*, a housekeeper, or a volunteer.' (Interview with Ms A, 13 November 2018)

This highlights the ambiguities that exist; it is hard to distinguish where the boundaries of official care and daily living assistance lie. What care service or daily life assistance should be covered by LTCIS? And how great a fee should the *Tsukisoifu* therefore charge the user?

Care work between employer and family

In caring work, it is not clear whether care for users should be undertaken as a paid job or conducted by volunteers or family members. A *Tsukisoifu* may care for the same person for many years. Since the *Tsukisoifu* spends a long time with users, they are sometimes in greater contact than the user's family. This can be illustrated by my own experience interviewing a *Tsukisoifu*.

I interviewed Ms A immediately after Ms B passed away. Ms A had been taking care of Ms B for more than ten years and was very shocked by the loss of Ms B. Ms A said that she lost her power and it felt like her whole body had gone. As mentioned earlier, Ms A had been making Ms B's favourite food at home and brought it to Ms B's home. Ms A continued to do it because she wanted to see Ms B's smiling face. When Ms B became able to eat from her mouth, her quality of life was improved. However, Ms A did not ask Ms B and her family to pay the cost, as she was pleased to make Ms B happy. When Ms B died, Ms A went to her funeral ceremony to say her final farewell. Ms A was invited to sit on the family seat by Ms B's family. Even after Ms B died, Ms A was asked by family members to come to Ms B's house to clean Ms B's room. Although Ms A was not family, there was an intimate relationship similar to a family, so a dilemma occurred. This highlights that the job of *Tsukisoifu* cannot be wholly business-like and it is difficult sometimes to request legitimate expense.

The work of CCWs, HVCWs and the *Tsukisoifu* therefore have complicated boundaries. The issues surrounding the boundaries that such care workers face is also pointed out in the UK (Saks and Allsop 2007) and Canada (Kelly and Bourgeault 2015), and are common to all countries with an ageing population. When care services are provided at the user's home, there is usually almost no oversight. And the decision on whether or not to work on or across the boundary may be left to the individual caregiver or follow the customs of the group to which the caregiver belongs. This is a different way of working from a health professional with certification and registration working in a more formal organisational setting in the public and private sectors, such as hospitals and nursing homes. It causes a greater possibility for risks to occur, on which there is further discussion in Chapter five.

Conclusion: who will play the role of carer?

How can we respond to the growing demand for health support workers as the ageing population accelerates? And who is expected to play this role? Elderly care is becoming more affordable after the implementation of the LTCIS, but it alone is not enough to support the lives of elderly people in Japan.

In order to make it easier to understand what kind of people might act as the main body of caregivers outside of medicine and nursing, I have categorised the types of care in Table 11.3 from the viewpoint of whether formal care (covered by LTCIS) or informal care (outside of LTCIS) occurs in social services or a privatised service.

To support the life of elderly people sustainably, an enhancement of formal care in social services may be needed. The Japanese government and its relevant authority (MHLW) have therefore given particular attention to two potential solutions: volunteers who are carrying out informal social services; and immigrant care workers.

Volunteers are now expected to be trained to support formal paid care. Approximately 1.2 million middle-aged people (50 to 64 years old) nationwide are now volunteering with the elderly – facilitated by, among others, the Welfare Human Resource Centre, Silver Human Resource Centre and the Volunteer Centre (Ministry of Health, Labor and Welfare Social Insurance Council 2017). In the caring field, inviting

Table 11.3: Structure of care services

	Formal care	Informal care
Social services	Social Worker Certified Care Worker Home Visiting Care Worker	Regional resources Social resources Unpaid carers and volunteers
Privatised service	Second opinion Paid rehabilitation therapy	*Tsukisoifu* Housekeeper

middle-aged people to volunteer is expected to help counteract the shortage of caregivers. The following actions may further support this:

- implementing introductory training and workplace experiences to learn the basic knowledge and skills necessary for engaging in care work; and
- supporting improvements (such as in workflow and the personnel management system) required of care providers when middle-aged people are accepted as volunteers.

In this way, an attempt is being made to create an opportunity for inexperienced volunteers to enter the caring field to address the anxiety that has become a barrier to entering the job market and to expand the range of care personnel available to the elderly. In the latest proposal, it was intended that the basic training would be evaluated in 2018 and started across the country from 2019 (MHLW 2017).

In recent years, the Japanese government has also tried to encourage the training and acceptance of foreign caregivers, such as in the roles of nurses and CCWs. Based on the Economic Partnership Agreement (EPA) with Indonesia, the Philippines and Vietnam, Japan has been accepting foreign nurses/care worker candidates since 2008 (MHLW 2018b). However, the national examination to obtain the CCW is very difficult: only 213 out of 420 candidates passed in 2018, giving a pass rate of 50.7 per cent (MHLW 2018c). In addition, even if the national exam is passed, there are many people who choose to return to their home country – in practice few actually stay in Japan and work as CCWs.

In terms of foreign nurse candidates, they are eligible to stay in Japan for three years before taking the national examination. Nurse candidates can take the national exam based on the EPA up to three times in total. However, at the first national examination in 2009, none passed out of 82 candidates. In 2010 only 3 out of 254 passed the examination. Eventually, in 2018, 78 out of 441 people (17.7 per cent) passed. It is therefore highly problematic for foreign students to pass the exam because of the need to master Japanese and understand the medical terms in the examination and health care legislation. Immigrant nurses and care workers who come to Japan therefore continue to face significant barriers. As a result, the Japanese government needs to improve the language training programme, create a rewarding workplace environment, and enhance the visa acquisiton process.

To protect the quality of life and wellbeing of elderly people, some other options can be proposed. One is to raise the LTCIS premium to extend formal care. Another is to let informal care workers do more work for the elderly. In addition, even in informal care, it is also possible to explore how social services could be shaped using the local social resources of volunteers and unpaid carers. In such cases, caring work should be made more attractive for individuals who have the potential to be care workers. Those adults who have finished raising a family or who have retired could be considered to be prime care work candidates. Such middle and old age care workers are a better option today, with ever more of the population living beyond the age of 100 (Gratton and Scott 2016). If such lay people are to increasingly come into the care field, more research-based evaluation is needed and the dynamics of professional dominance should be reconsidered.

All countries must respond the demographic trend of ageing. The Japanese challenge is particularly great at present, so it is an important example to consider in relation to future policy effectiveness. While many developed countries have at least some policies in place for the care of the elderly, most developing countries are unprepared for the challenge of ageing (Shetty 2012). Yet their populations may become old before they become rich enough to be able to prepare. As Peterson (1999:55) says: 'We must establish new ways of thinking and new institutions to help us prepare for a much older world.' At the heart of this is providing and preparing sufficient cohorts of both paid support workers and unpaid carers and volunteers at all levels to mitigate what can be seen as an ever more pressing crisis situation.

References

Akeno, N., Hatakeyama, M., Fujimoto, S., and Ishikawa, K. (2017) 'Actual conditions relating to the implementation of glycerin enema and faeces at a Visiting Nursing Care Center', *Bulletin of the Faculty of Nursing and Welfare*, Hokkaido Medical University 24: 23–29.

Arai, T. (1991) *Looking at a Number of Deaths*, Tokyo: Asahi–Bunko Publisher.

Gratton, L. and Scott, A. (2016) *The 100-Year Life*, London: Bloomsbury.

Hosoda, M. (2012) *What Is Team Medicine?* Tokyo: Japan Nursing Association.

Japan Medical Association (1999) *Japanese Doctor News* 914, 5 October.

Japan Nursing Association (1993) *Hospital Nursing Basic Survey 1991: Research Report 39*, Tokyo: JNA.

Japan Nursing Association (2016) *Ministry of Health, Labor and Welfare Health Service Promotion Fees and Other Subsidies: Business Research Report on the Role Required of Nursing Staff in Nursing Facilities*, Tokyo: JNA.

Kelly, C. and Bourgeault, I. (2015) 'The personal support worker program standard in Ontario: An alternative to self-regulation?', *Healthcare Policy* 11(2): 20–26.

Ministry of Health, Labor and Welfare (MHLW) (2013) *Survey of Nursing Labour Situation in 2008 Fiscal Year, 2012 Nursing Care Service Facility Establishment Survey and 2013 Year Wage Structure Basic Statistical Survey*, Tokyo: MHLW.

MHLW (2016) *Trends in Number of Care Worker Registered Persons*, Tokyo: MHLW.

MHLW (2017) *Annual Health Welfare Report 2017: Health and Welfare Services for the Elderly*, www.mhlw.go.jp/english/wp/wp-hw11/dl/10e.pdf

MHLW (2018a) *Outline of Ministry of Health, Labor and Welfare: Care Worker*, www.mhlw.go.jp/kouseiroudoushou/shikaku_shiken/kaigohukushishi/

MHLW (2018b) *Acceptance of Foreign Nurses and Care Worker Candidates from Indonesia, Philippines and Vietnam*, www.mhlw.go.jp/stf/seisakunitsuite/bunya/koyou_roudou/koyou/gaikokujin/other22/index.html

MHLW (2018c) *The Result of the 30th CCW National Examination*, www.mhlw.go.jp/file/04-Houdouhappyou-12004000-Shakaiengokyoku-Shakai-Fukushikibanka/0000199589.pdf

Ministry of Health, Labor and Welfare Social Insurance Council (2017) *Long-Term Care Benefit Expense Sub-committee*, 23 August, www.wic-net.com/pdftmp/3088_1_3_1548421571.pdf#page=1

Mizuho Information and Research Institute (2012) *Survey Study on Problems and Support Policies of Elderly People and Elderly Households Living Alone, 2011 Report*, Tokyo: MIRI.

National Institute of Population and Social Security Research (2017) *Population Projections for Japan: 2016–2065,* Population Research Series No. 336.

Ohnishi, G. and Ohnishi, Y. (2009) 'Case study of medical incident: Lifesaving with AED', *Clinical Journal of Imabari Medical Association* 12: 52–3.

Okamoto, Y., Tsujimura, M., Yoshinaga, A., Ota, S. and Ishigaki, K. (2006) 'Research on defecation assistance by visiting nurse to elderly people who need long-term care and suffer from bowel movement and family caregivers who cannot help defecation', *Journal of the Chiba Nursing Association* 12(1): 100–107.

Peterson, P. (1999) 'Gray dawn: The global aging crisis', *Foreign Affairs* 78(1): 42–55.

Saks, M. (2010) 'Analyzing the professions: The case for the neo-Weberian approach', *Comparative Sociology* 9(6): 887–915.

Saks, M. (2016) 'Professions and power', in Dent, M., Bourgeault, I., Dennis, J. and Kuhlmann, E. (eds) *The Routledge Companion to the Professions and Professionalism,* Abingdon: Routledge.

Saks, M. and Allsop, J. (2007) 'Social policy, professional regulation and health support work in the United Kingdom', *Social Policy and Society* 6(2): 165–77.

Sasaki, M. and Takiuchi, T. (2009) 'Practice situation of nursing constipation and future subjects', *Bulletin of the Department of Health Sciences,* Graduate School of Medicine, Akita University 17(2): 37–43.

Shetty, P. (2012) 'Grey matter', *Lancet* 379:1285–87.

Shinozaki, R. (2002) *How Far Is It Permitted? The Medical Practice of Home Helpers,* Tokyo: Hitotsubashi Publishing.

Shinozaki, R. (2005) 'The actual condition of medical care by care workers and the effects of their training', Medical Safety Promoter Network (medsafe), www.medsafe.net/contents/recent/81helper.html

Shinozaki, R. (2008) 'Medical practice of nursing career: Do you really want the site?', *Monthly Care Management* 20(1): 62–5.

Shiraishi, T. (2013) 'Adverse event investigation and safety assessment of glycerin enema', *Medicine and Pharmacy* 69(1): 97–100.

Sugiyama, A. (1995) *Medical Reform in the Occupied Period in Japan,* Tokyo: Keisu Shobo Publisher.

Zarit, S., Todd, P. and Zarit, J. (1986) 'Subjective burden of husbands and wives as caregivers: A longitudinal study', *The Gerontologist* 26(3): 260–66.

World Health Organization (2019) 'Ageing and Life Course', www.who.int/ageing/en/

Index

Printed and bound by CPI Group (UK) Ltd, Croydon, CR0 4YY

16/04/2025

14658340-0003

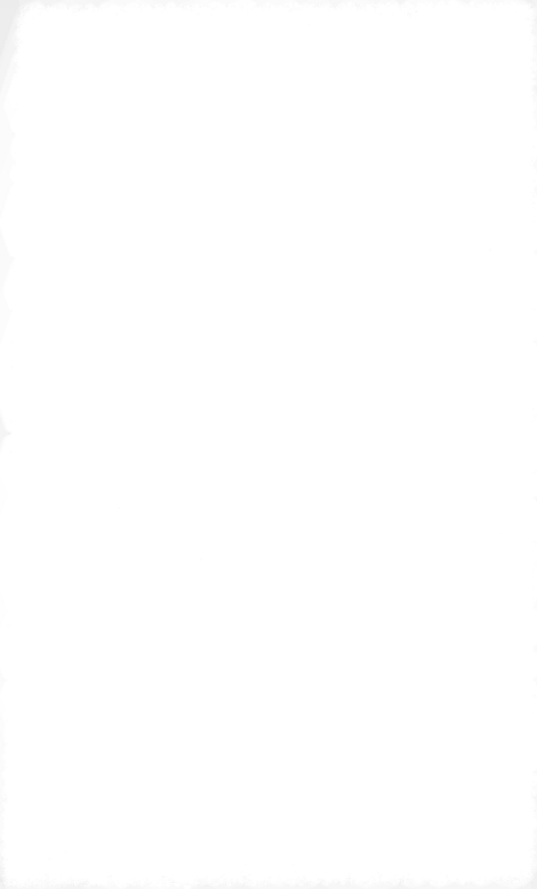

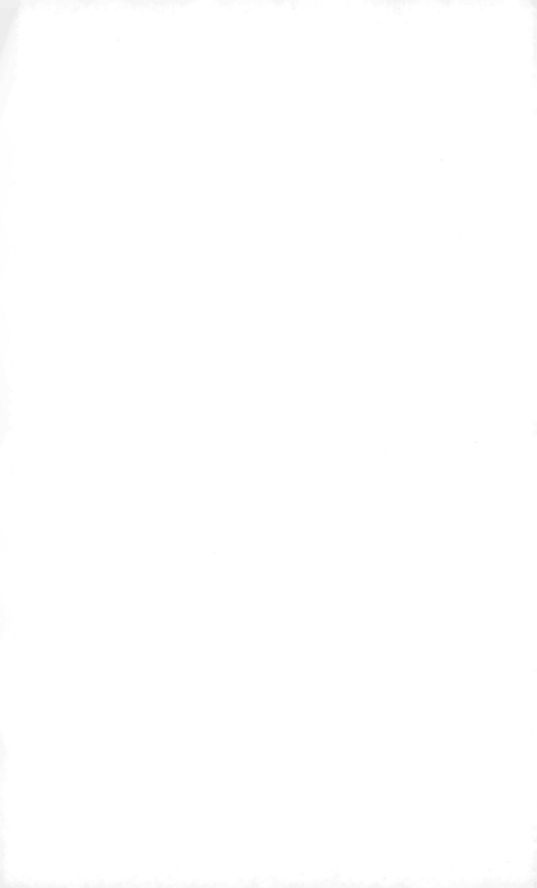